Praise for Hope & Healing: The Case for Cannabis

"Insightful and thought-provoking. I do admire his tenacity to serve his patients, at not being scared off by the politics or road bumps. It shows his drive, it shows he's a leader and an innovator. Bravo for facing the tough stuff!"

—Diane D. Rodriguez
Grief Educator, Bereavement Coach & Consultant, Writer & Speaker

"Very well researched and an easy and entertaining read. A person with no knowledge about medical cannabis will be illuminated after reading *Hope & Healing* by Dr. Rosado. I hope many people will be reached with the knowledge Dr. Rosado is sharing. Congratulations on a very interesting text!"

—Juan Camilo Jaramillo
Marine Biologist

"Hats off to Dr. Rosado and for the work he's doing. I appreciated and enjoyed much of the book, especially the early portions where he describes the history and background, noting how it came to be that cannabis is considered a dangerous substance rather than a potential healing intervention. The book seems to be aimed at potential patients who may have some hesitation to pursue medical cannabis, and for that audience, I think those sections would be appealing."

—DAVID SACKS, PH.D.
Psychologist, Writer

"During the first 15 years of my career, I was in law enforcement where it was drilled into my head that marijuana is bad, period. However, now as a writer specializing in natural health and wellness, I've read numerous studies that say the complete opposite. This begs to question: who's right? What I love most about this book is that Dr. Rosado provides an answer that is simple and in an easy-to-read manner. Plus, it is chock full of information that I've never known, such as how the negative stigma associated with marijuana actually began. (I've researched and written about this topic several times before and never have I seen this explained so well!) As a result, I now have a clearer idea as to why this particular drug has been blackballed, as well as the numerous obstacles it has yet to overcome. Additionally, this book has really opened my eyes to the real-life benefits cannabis has to offer. That is, if we just give it a chance."

—CHRISTINA DEBUSK
Health and Wellness Writer, Editor, Speaker

HOPE &
HEALING

The Case for Cannabis

HOPE &

HEALING

The Case for Cannabis

Cancer | Epilepsy and Seizures | Glaucoma
HIV and AIDS | Crohn's Disease
Chronic Muscle Spasms and Multiple Sclerosis
PTSD | ALS | Parkinson's Disease
Chronic Pain | Other Ailments

DR. JOSEPH ROSADO, M.D.
with Rodney Miles and a Foreword by
Professor Lumír Ondřej Hanuš

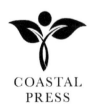

COASTAL
PRESS

For information about special discounts for bulk purchases or author interviews, appearances, and speaking engagements please contact:

Dr. Joseph Rosado, M.D.
www.JosephRosadoMD.com
info@josephrosadomd.com
1 (866) 763-7991

First Edition

ISBNs
978-1-946875-34-1 hardcover
978-1-946875-35-8 paperback
978-1-946875-36-5 ebook
Kindle ASIN: B07QYQJMLR
Amazon paperback: ISBN-13: 978-1687506528

Edited, book and cover design by Rodney Miles: www.RodneyMiles.com

For all who hope to heal

"Science is the father of knowledge, but opinion breeds ignorance."

—HIPPOCRATES

CONTENTS

A NOTE TO READERS

"Healing is a matter of time, but it is sometimes also a matter of opportunity."

—HIPPOCRATES
Greek Philosopher and Physician
Called "The Father of Medicine"

THIS BOOK was written to fill a void too often experienced by those of you who might have wondered about the usefulness of cannabis as treatment. It is intended for a lay audience, and while I do explore some of the science in *Hope & Healing*, it was always intended and written with you—presumably a non-expert—in mind. I find bookstores (online and otherwise) are more and more filled with books about cannabis but

xvi

they are usually intended for a recreational-use audience eager for news on broad legalization. But interestingly, cannabis is not my "drug of choice."

I have arrived where I am today in my passions and in my profession by the hard facts which are often obfuscated or maligned in a continuing—if declining—resignation to see the use of cannabis prevented. For that reason, as with any "extended black propaganda campaign," as in the case of cannabis, we can stand to be disabused of many previously held "facts," and find correct ones to put in their place. This needs to be done even before a discussion of the science behind medicinal cannabis can be undertaken, therefore we do this in the beginning of *Hope & Healing.* Only then do we follow with informal discussions of the current science, laws, and things you can do to benefit from medicinal cannabis.

Both the science and the laws are sure to evolve, even in the brief period between the final draft and actual release of this book. Cannabis as a subject and as a science is quickly developing all over the world. Tipping points are being reached. Therefore, assuming your interest in the subject, I recommend you stay abreast of laws in your state as well as the growing availability of medicinal cannabis and the likely burgeoning local resources. In some cases, people travel far or even relocate in the interest of their health or the health and well-being of a loved one. You might also connect with me, of course, through my contact information in the back of this book.

I am a physician based in Florida and use Florida in all examples and explanations of legal, medical use of cannabis within the State. (All referenced sources are listed at the end of the book, in the "Notes" section.) Across the United States and across the world cannabis is, as I write this, becoming more accepted, considered, recommended, and legalized. While the full legalization of medicinal cannabis seems inevitable, there are minds and laws to change, and this explains what delays might still exist, for there are often not moral nor ethical arguments preventing its broad acceptance, but legal ones. States simply wait to see what happens in other states before proceeding "too quickly." Any reader on the subject will soon discover this.

In your case, or in the case of a loved one, you might not have time to wait nor time to waste in seeking the most effective, generally side-effect-free remedies available. This book is for you, and while Florida is used in my story and in my examples, always consult local laws and your own medical professionals before proceeding with cannabis or any medical remedy.

No matter where you are, there is *hope* and there can be *healing,* for the laws of God and Nature trump the laws of man, every time.

FOREWORD

By Professor Lumír Ondřej Hanuš

"If patients are to have a humane right to health, they would have full access to this medicinal plant. There are plenty of cases where cannabis is a patient's only hope."

—LUMÍR HANUŠ

IF YOU SAY, "carry coals to Newcastle," or "bring sand to the beach," that is exactly what I mean if we shall talk about the history of the recreational, industrial, or medicinal use of the famous plant called *Cannabis sativa* (also *hemp* or *cannabis*). It is a plant used by humankind for millennia. This history is today notoriously known, so let me acquaint you with its medical history in Olomouc, that unknown city in the world today where after the stigmatization, a modern rebirth of medicinal cannabis occurred.

In 1950 during a study of higher plants for antibiotic principles, professor Zdeněk Krejčí discovered at Palacký University (within the City of Olomouc in Czechoslovakia) that Cannabis sativa has significant antibacterial effects upon gram-positive microorganisms including some common pathogenic microorganisms. It was immediately and successfully examined clinically (stomatology, otorhinolaryngology, gynecology, dermatology, etc.) and in time for a scientific conference on "Hemp as a Medicine" to be held on December 10, 1954 (on Human Rights Day). That conference was held in Olomouc. (You must understand that any Cannabis sativa is in the fact *hemp,* even when today it is used only for the strain used for fibers). All lectures from this conference were published as scientific papers at Palacký University Acta and one can find these studies today online at http://www.bushka.cz/KabelikEN/index.html.

Professor Krejčí together with Professor František Šantavý succeeded in isolating and identifying the compound responsible for this antibacterial effect and named it *cannabidiolic acid* (published in 1955). In fact, it was the first known real cannabinoid, as within the plant all cannabinoids are in the form of their cannabinoid acids. It was the first modern use of cannabis as a medicine. Since that time in Olomouc, cannabis has been used at Faculty Hospital for treatment (on the level of the knowledge of that time) up to 1990 when I left to do research at Hebrew University in Jerusalem.

While a "witch hunt" took place in the U.S. in connection with cannabis (shouted most loudly by those who apparently did not know anything about cannabis), at the hospital in Czechoslovakia we treated patients with cannabis which had a *CBD to THC ratio* (expressed CBD:THC) of approximately 4:1, and this happened between the years of 1954 and 1990. After my departure cannabis unfortunately became an illegal plant in Czechoslovakia. However, cannabis research after 1954 has continued.

In 1963, through research independent of each other, Professor Šantavý in Czechoslovakia and Professors Mechoulam and Shvo in Israel elucidated the structure of cannabidiol (CBD), and in 1964 Šantavý in Czechoslovakia, and independent of him, Gaoni and Mechoulam in Israel elucidated the structure of (-)-trans-9-tetrahydrocannabinol (THC). In 1988 when William Devane discovered central cannabinoid receptors (CB1) in the brain, the role of THC in the organism was explained. The most recent advance was in 1992 when on March 24, after my last purification (of substances) I had in my own hands the pure compound, ligand, which is a natural compound in the human brain (we later named it *anandamide*), which binds to the CB1 receptor. Finally, after a millennia of medical use of cannabis, we reached a scientific explanation, and from that time we have observed a virtual explosion of scientific research and medicinal uses of cannabis around the globe. Although research is expanding exponentially today, we are still only at the beginning of a full understanding of cannabis treatment.

Cannabis is not a miraculous plant, it is not a panacea. But cannabinoid receptors are some of the most widely spread in the human body, and that is why it works with so many diseases. It is reasonable that in the near future it will treat *almost all diseases at least palliatively.* I previously never supported the full legalization of cannabis, but it now seems this may be the only effective way to ensure full treatment of patients. At present time, patients are rather hostages of their treatment, as they do not have access to sufficient amounts nor correct strains of cannabis to treat their diseases. Often they do not have enough on hand not only for curative use but not even for palliative uses.

It should be clear that cannabis is one of the safest medicines in the world and there is no reason to prohibit it. It is dangerous only for companies that stand to lose income by introducing cannabis into healthcare. There are very few patients who cannot be treated with cannabis, who do not feel good after its use or who it does not help. Even in these cases, it's possible they took too big a dose (were overdosed) or used an incorrect strain of cannabis. Sometimes they must try several strains to they find the correct one. Unfortunately, not every patient has the opportunity or access to try different strains. But even *overdose* is not harmful, if uncomfortable. In fact, for a mentally healthy adult person, cannabis is not harmful, even with long-term use.

Marijuana is not a completely benign substance. It is a powerful drug with a variety of effects. However, except for the harms associated with smoking, the adverse effects of marijuana use are within the range of effects tolerated for other medications. Throughout the therapeutic use of cannabis, it is necessary to identify not only the patients who can benefit from its use, but also those whom it may harm! It seems quite clear, however, that the risk is much higher in children and adolescents (particularly before puberty). Both doctors and parents will continue to face the difficult decision whether to treat youngsters with this plant and hope that it will cause greater good than harm. It may be assumed that cannabis can damage the adolescent brain, but not—in contrast to alcohol—the adult brain. Important risks include triggering of psychosis, schizophrenia, and cognitive impairments (usually worsening short-term memory). Thankfully, most adolescents who abuse marijuana do not become psychotic adults.

If patients are to have a humane right to health, they would have full access to this medicinal plant. There are plenty of cases where cannabis is a patient's only hope. I hope that in the near future the power of this plant will be fully known and accessible worldwide, for any patient, whether rich or poor. God in nature created this healing plant *for you,* the patient, so that you might recover from your disease with the help of this amazing plant, and that is why I am now for the full legalization of cannabis—not because of recreational users but because of cannabis patients. Legalization now seems necessary just to guarantee patients the patient correct amount and chemotype (equivalent to strain, cultivar, variety, chemovar) which can help them.

This book is part of making the power of cannabis as a medicine fully known. Because of my research activities, I generally do not have time to read books, but when I started to read *Hope & Healing,* I read it with bated breath and could not stop until I finished a whole reading. This is really a very good book, which I can suggest to both specialists as well as "ordinary" readers. It's a book full of important information regarding certain diseases and their possible treatment by cannabis. Evaluate the information in this book for yourself. I shall definitely keep it in my library for now and the future.

—LUMÍR HANUŠ
Jerusalem, December 10, 2018
on Human Rights Day

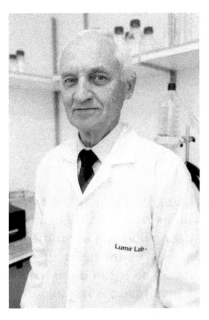

PROFESSOR LUMÍR ONDŘEJ HANUŠ is a world-renowned analytical chemist and a leading figure in the field of cannabis research. He is responsible for groundbreaking and award-winning research in the world of cannabinoids and his research serves as the basis for much of what we know about the plant today. Professor Hanuš isolated the first known endocannabinoid in the human brain, Anandamide, named after the Sanskrit word for bliss. The discovery of Anandamide confirmed that the human brain produces "cannabinoids" of its own, called endocannabinoids, which bind with cannabinoid receptors throughout the brain and body. Evidence suggests these cannabinoid receptors are involved in neuroprotection, pain modulation, memory processing, motor coordination, control of appetite, and more. Since Professor Hanuš' immense discovery, thousands of studies have been conducted on the endocannabinoid system and on cannabinoids of all kinds. This transformative revelation has affected and more importantly shaped the industry as we now know it. Meanwhile, additional cannabinoids from plant, and endocannabinoids from humans and other living organisms, continue to be discovered.

Professor Lumír Ondřej Hanuš. Image © 2018 Lumir Lab

"The evidence is overwhelming that marijuana can relieve certain types of pain, nausea, vomiting and other symptoms caused by such illnesses as multiple sclerosis, cancer and AIDS — or by the harsh drugs sometimes used to treat them. And it can do so with remarkable safety. Indeed, marijuana is less toxic than many of the drugs that physicians prescribe every day."

—DR. JOYCELYN ELDERS, MD,
Former U.S. Surgeon General
March 26, 2004, "Myths About Medical Marijuana,"
Providence Journal

INTRODUCTION: THE ART OF HEALING

"The art of healing comes from nature, not from the physician. Therefore, the physician must start from nature, with an open mind."

—PARACELSUS
Swiss Physician, Alchemist, and
Astrologer of the German Renaissance

EVER SINCE I was three years old, I wanted to be a medical doctor. I was born in 1962 in Manhattan and raised in the Bronx, and back then the obstetricians used to take care of the kids for the first few years. They would perform the well-child visits and administer the vaccines and so on. But it got to the point that I developed, at a very young age, PTSD. My mother would be carrying me to the doctor's office and the *instant* I saw the street block or something I recognized I began to scream. I *did not* want to be there. And our obstetrician didn't do appointments, it was first-come, first-serve. He had a list, the moms would sign their names on the list, and you would be there for *hours.* It was ridiculous. But thanks to my continual resistance it got to the point where this doctor told my mother, "Look, you're going to have to find a pediatrician. I can't continue with this (my fits) any longer."

"Who do you recommend?" she asked.

"There's a Doctor Romero, a pediatrician I work with at the hospital," he said. "When I deliver babies, he's there to take care of them. You may want to try him." And it turned out that individual was a distant cousin of a friend of our family, so we went to his office. Because the office was new to me, it wasn't as traumatic for me, but as soon as we got into the actual office, with the familiar sights, the smells, the exam table, the stethoscope and the familiar medical equipment in there, I became hyper, I started crying. My parents were at either side of me and he was in front of me. My parents were trying to console me.

"Leave him alone," Doctor Romero said.

Now, that was weird to me, because whenever I went to the other guy, it was always, "Hold him down!"

It got my attention when this new doctor said that. *Hmm,* I thought, *There's something here. This is different!* At three years old, you can't put true meanings to things, but it was like something new and different had just happened. Then he said the magic words.

"Examine *me*," he said.

He put the otoscope[1] in my one hand and the tongue depressor in my other. He squatted down and he said again, "Examine me."

My parents then said, "Go ahead, examine him!" And I was linked, right then and there. In fact, the instant I felt those instruments in my hands, there was some type of cellular memory. *This is familiar to me,* I thought, *this is comfortable.* And that was it, from that point forward I knew I was going to be a medical doctor.

I would take the long road.

At five years old I developed very bad allergies and I had to go to Doctor Romero's office every week for a shot in each arm. I would show up with my mom and we'd sit there and wait until he'd take us in and give me my shots, and we'd walk away. No crying, no more drama, nothing. At the age of 15 I took an orderly course while in high school. When I turned 16 I worked as an orderly at an assisted living facility (nursing home). I transferred to Florida Hospital and worked as a transportation orderly in the x-ray department, then worked as an orderly again in 1984 in the post-anesthesia care unit (recovery room). And by then I was an emergency medical technician (EMT), so I had gone from orderly to EMT, and from EMT I became a paramedic. From paramedic, I became a heart catheterization lab technician. I then went to chiropractic school, and then to medical school.

I was initially exposed to the facts about cannabis in medical school, in the pharmacology class. We learned a lot of the different medications, their side-effects, and so on. And it was there that I learned from the textbooks of pharmacology that there were *no adverse reactions* to the use of cannabis and that there was technically *no lethal dose.* Therefore, the possibility and the probability of

---

[1] An instrument for examining the interior of the ear, especially the eardrum, consisting essentially of a magnifying lens and a light —The American Heritage Stedman's Medical Dictionary

addiction and of overdose was *non-existent*. Even today we discuss how cannabis has a psychological dependence but not a physiological dependence or addiction. Whether you smoke one or ten joints, the effect is technically going to be the same, contrary to cocaine or opiates, where you have to constantly increase the dose. That's where everything started for me, and after medical school, I got an MBA in healthcare management.

In 2010, when medical cannabis became legal in Arizona, one of my very good friends reached out to me about the possibility of working together, and my being the medical director at the dispensary. In Arizona the law states that every dispensary has to have an M.D. (medical doctor or "allopathic" doctor) or D.O. (osteopathic doctor) or naturopath overseeing the dispensary. We were all set to move forward, but at the time, these friends had a teenage son who was one or two weeks older than my twin daughters, and they decided because they wished to promote abstinence when it came to recreational drugs, the plan was not going to be a good thing for them and they decided not to move forward.

I moved back to Florida in 2009, began practicing medicine there, and by late 2012 I was starting to *burn out*. I was in a group practice, on call in the ER every other day where I consulted, admitted, and followed my own patients in a community hospital in Levy County, Florida. I was the medical director of the same community hospital and was also the medical director for a home health agency. I was in a practice that had multiple HMO contracts and *every day* we had no fewer than 37 patients scheduled. Management wanted to be certain we saw at least 30 patients per day, so in the event of no-shows or cancellations, I could still "make the quota."

Physicians in recent years have been notoriously frustrated by being both overworked and underpaid by the insurance industry, often seeing at least 25 patients per day just to break even. Many experience *burnout*, which is defined as a loss of enthusiasm for work, feelings of cynicism, and a low sense of personal accomplishment. In fact, burnout among U.S. physicians has reached a critical level. In a recent Medscape report, the highest percentages of burnout occurred in critical care, urology, and emergency medicine, all at *55 percent*. Family medicine and internal medicine follow closely at 54 percent. The 2015 survey published in the Mayo Clinic Proceedings compared burnout between 2011 and 2014 and observed an *increase* in the percentage of physicians reporting at least one burnout symptom, from 45.5 percent to 54.4 percent. It was, in general, getting worse. I wanted more for myself and more for my patients.

Then, in the spring of 2014, I saw the TV ads with Florida attorney John Morgan regarding Amendment 2[2], which stirred up that whole desire in me again to find and administer a side-effect-free and efficacious remedy for patients. I began to learn more about medical cannabis. I purchased the *Handbook of Cannabis* and approached my learning with the same attitude as when I was studying for my boards. As I read and studied, I attended seminars put on by the Florida Cannabis Coalition, and researched physicians in Colorado and Maine and attended their seminars, all in preparation for the eventual decriminalization of medical cannabis in Florida.

I continued learning, studying and preparing, and in 2015, I enrolled in and received the certification from the Florida Department of Health to recommend high-CBD/low-THC under Senate Bill 1030, also called the Compassionate Care Act, in the hopes that it would position me in a place where I could phase out of primary

---

[2] The Florida Medical Marijuana Legalization Initiative, also called "Amendment 2," passed in Florida on November 8th, 2016, approving the use of cannabis for medical purposes. We discuss this in greater detail throughout the book.

care and transition into a medical cannabis practice. With certification in 2015, the passing of Amendment 2 in 2016 and its taking effect in January of 2017, I have evolved into a place where approximately 65 percent of my practice is dedicated to seeing Compassionate Care and medical cannabis patients.

There is no insurance coverage (yet) for the recommending of medical cannabis, therefore, it's a cash practice. The patients are appreciative of obtaining a "medication" they have longed to receive for years—in fact, I have yet to have a patient ask for insulin or "more pills," but my medical cannabis patients are always eager for their medical cannabis cards. There is great personal gratification in providing a service that is sorely needed and too rarely provided. Less than one percent of Florida's 55,000 doctors currently hold licenses to order medical cannabis. In South Florida, about 150 have licenses, according to the state database. But even those with a license are being cautious about ordering medical cannabis.

We can all agree that the number of people on pain medications, tranquilizers, anxiety pills, and sleeping pills in this state is staggering and the side-effects are more dangerous than medical cannabis. My position is if I can take a person who is dying and help them improve their well-being, help them enjoy food, help decrease the aches and pains of dying, then what I'm doing is a blessing, and I've been consistently told as much by the hundreds of patients I am currently seeing for medical cannabis. And it all happens while helping people live better lives and making the world a better place.

It made me think about Doctor Romero, my childhood doctor who had turned the table on me and let me examine *him*. It's about what works. It's all about "do no harm." Dr. Romero was truly an amazing human being. In fact, as of four or five years ago he was still practicing in a community clinic in Harlem, New York, as a pediatrician. When I called and introduced myself to the office staff, I said, "Hi, I was a former patient of Dr. Romero when I was a child until the age of 15. I'm a physician now, and I'd like to speak with him and let him know that he made a huge impact in my life."

"We'll leave him a message," she said.

"Thank you. Out of curiosity, is he still a tall, distinguished man, with a deep voice?"

"Completely," she said.

"He was my pediatrician," I said, and I went on with all of the people I knew he had serviced in the City of New York.

Today I am a licensed, primary care physician and I'm an advocate for the medicinal use of cannabis in the state of Florida. I participated in the United for Care campaign during the 2014 and 2016 elections in Florida. I've completed the state required eight-hour course on recommending high-CBD:low-THC cannabis for medicinal use. I've completed the two-hour medical director course. I have taken the two-hour course on recommending high-CBD:low-THC and medical cannabis. I've recommended low-THC and medical cannabis with, at this writing, over 1,000 patients. I was the first in Florida (Central Florida) to recommend, in the summer of 2016, low-THC:high-CBD cannabis, and in the fall of 2016, the first to recommend 1:1 (THC:CBD) in Florida for a terminal child. I guess you could say I am a pioneer. I have the scars to prove it, and the happy patients.

But this book, more than being about me, the law, or even medical cannabis, is rather about *hope*. I wrote it because I want to show you in very simple terms *why and how* medical cannabis works, and from my own experience as a practicing physician, how it might just help you. When you can see that, you will see why I have decided to take the harder road in mainstream medicine, why I've chosen to take the slings of a pioneer in this field. But I can't do that until we address at least some of the concerns you might have about "medical marijuana," many of which are simply created out of thin air, created out of fear and ignorance with no basis in fact, historically for a political or even a racist basis. You might be shocked.

Are *you* or someone you love a potential cannabis patient and don't know if your condition qualifies for medical cannabis under Florida law? Do you have questions about what physicians can and cannot do in the State of Florida when it comes to medical marijuana? Do you have questions about what medical cannabis is, the forms it's available in, the state of legality in Florida, or if there are benefits and side-effects you are not aware of? Are you wondering how the whole process works?

Let's start with the word itself, "marijuana." It very likely doesn't mean what you think it does.

"In strict medical terms marijuana is far safer than many foods we commonly consume. For example, eating 10 raw potatoes can result in a toxic response. By comparison, it is physically impossible to eat enough marijuana to induce death. Marijuana in its natural form is one of the safest therapeutically active substances known to man. By any measure of rational analysis marijuana can be safely used within the supervised routine of medical care."

—Hon. Francis Young
DEA Administrative Law Judge
Ruling in the matter of "Marijuana Rescheduling Petition," September 6, 1988

PART I: CONTROVERSY

[1] REEFER MADNESS

> "All propaganda has to be popular and has to accommodate itself to the comprehension of the least intelligent of those whom it seeks to reach."
>
> —ADOLF HITLER
> Leader of the Nazi Party (from 1920/21),
> Chancellor and Führer of Germany (1933–45)

ON HIS FIRST day in office, August 12, 1930, Harry J. Anslinger had a problem. He was accustomed to notoriety and he was ambitious. Born in 1892 into the stern morality of the Victorian era, by the age of 23 he had made a name for himself as a young investigator for the Pennsylvania Railroad. He had proved a widower's $50,000 claim as a fraud, saving the company thousands, making a name for himself, and earning a promotion to captain of railroad police. He then traveled the world with various police and military organizations and returned to the U.S. in 1929 as an assistant commissioner in the Treasury Department's Bureau of Prohibition. During prohibition, Anslinger seemed to have no beef with cannabis, claiming it was not harmful nor did it incite violence. But the war on alcohol was failing, and the Department of Prohibition, of which he was now in charge, was becoming obsolete.

So, in 1930 when he was appointed as the first commissioner of the Federal Bureau of Narcotics by his wife's uncle, he knew he needed a *cause*. And over the next seven years—coincident with the rise of the DuPont (chemical) and Hearst (media) empires—Anslinger had decided, ostensibly, that his new agency's mission would be the suppression of cannabis (often called "Indian hemp" in government documents up until the 1940s). He would make the Bureau—and himself—significant again. And he did. Over the next 30 years he would establish the global headquarters for the "war on drugs," an effort that today consumes over $51 *billion dollars* annually in the United States alone.

UP UNTIL 1910 the word "marijuana" had not been used broadly in the United States. Instead, "cannabis" was used, and generally in reference to medicines and remedies for common ailments. Drug companies also included cannabis and its extracts in certain medicines. But what was popular among American elites (especially literary elites) was *hashish*, a resin extracted from cannabis that holds psychoactive ingredients. Beginning in 1910 (and through 1920, the years of the Mexican Revolution), almost one million Mexicans legally immigrated to the U.S., taking refuge from the devastation of the war and expanding the popularity of cannabis as a recreational form of cigarette.

The first resistance came in a 1913 bill that criminalized cultivation of "locoweed" in California, with the support of the Board of Pharmacy—not in an effort to ban it, but rather in an effort to regulate opiates and pharmaceuticals.

The United States then plunged into the Great Depression, when jobs became dangerously rare. Many (mostly whites) would start to resent the large number of immigrants and minorities in the country in the struggle for jobs, and many would start to resent the rise of jazz and other cultural changes and associate the smoking of cannabis with corruption of both mind and body.

The rise of the word, "marijuana" is still debated today, but theories include its invention as a racial slur against the Mexican and other immigrants of the day, derived from either the Mexican-Spanish term "marihuana" (with an "h") which may derive from the Aztec "mallihuan," which means "prisoner," or the Chinese "ma ren hua," which means "hemp seed flower," or possibly from the Spanish "mejorana" or English "marjoram," meaning oregano. The association with the personal name "Mary Jane" is likely folklore.

"Marijuana," with a "j" is an Americanized version of the word and rose in use in the 1930s, a period rife with new popularity and debate over use of the substance, so much so that this was the word used as new laws were passed and new propaganda pushed to associate cannabis with the lower classes.

One of the foremost individuals engaged in creating stigma around cannabis in the 1930s and beyond was, of course, Harry Anslinger. As part of the campaign he initiated to stigmatize and racialize the plant for mostly white audiences, Anslinger placed messages in movie theaters across the country. He even made the following statement before Congress in 1937:

"Marijuana is the most violence-causing drug in the history of mankind ... Most (marijuana smokers) are Negroes, Hispanics, Filipinos and entertainers. Their Satanic music, jazz and swing, result from marijuana use. This marijuana causes white women to seek sexual relations with Negroes, entertainers, and any others."

He is also famous for the now-unthinkable statement:

"Reefer makes darkies think they're as good as white men ... the primary reason to outlaw marijuana is its effect on the degenerate races."

Anslinger also played a role in the creation of that now ridiculous yet seminal propaganda piece, *Reefer Madness,* filmed in 1936 and released in 1938, which depicts the tragedy and insanity that befalls misled teenagers lured into the use of marijuana. All along, the use of a "foreign sounding" term for cannabis clearly seems to have intentionally played upon the xenophobia of the age. Witness this promotional material from *Reefer Madness:*

"FOREWORD: The motion picture you are about to witness may startle you. It would not have been possible, otherwise, to sufficiently emphasize the frightful toll of the new drug menace which is destroying the youth of America in alarmingly-increasing numbers. Marihuana is that drug - a violent narcotic - an unspeakable scourge - The Real Public Enemy Number One! Its first effect is sudden, violent, uncontrollable laughter; then come dangerous hallucinations - space expands - time slows down, almost stands still . . . fixed ideas come next, conjuring up monstrous extravagances - followed by emotional disturbances, the total inability to direct thoughts, the loss of all power to resist physical emotions... leading finally to acts of shocking violence... ending often in incurable insanity. In picturing its soul-destroying effects no attempt was made to equivocate. The scenes and incidents, while fictionized for the purposes of this story, are based upon actual research into the results of Marihuana addiction. If their stark reality will make you think, will make you aware that something must be done to wipe out this ghastly menace, then the picture will not have failed in its purpose . . . Because the dread Marihuana may be reaching forth next for your son or daughter . . . or yours . . . or YOURS!"

Today *Reefer Madness* is universally recognized as classic propaganda, ridiculous hyperbole, but it had a lasting effect, it created a stigma or at least a doubt that still exists in degrees and in places today. The film suggests cannabis use—which up until recent years had been mainly medicinal—leads to any number of calamities:

- Hit and run incidents
- Manslaughter
- Suicide
- Rape
- Hallucinations

- Madness

Reefer Madness was originally financed by a church group and titled *Tell Your Children* but discovered and purchased by producer Dwain Esper, then distributed as an exploitation film. Today it has gained new popularity, as *satire*.

WHILE HARRY ANSLINGER would continue his all-out war on cannabis for thirty years, his first big victory came with the passage of the *Marihuana Tax Act of 1937*. It was the first big step to complete prohibition and made a crime out of the cultivation and use of cannabis all across the United States. Anslinger played a major role at the Department of Prohibition. Reports from the 1920s which claimed a decrease in drug use thanks to the war on drugs were found by historian David Courtwright through a Freedom of Information Act request to have been fabricated, and Anslinger himself admitted in a private memo the "numbers were made up." Yet he used these fabrications to expand the drug war to include cannabis. Regardless of his inner beliefs, Harry Anslinger clearly used racism to demonize cannabis, and he lied to suit his cause and glorify his position and importance.

And the now infamous "war on drugs" was officially underway. Years later, it would seem the perfect political opportunity, and be expanded by yet another political official, one who ended his political career in disgrace.

[2] TRICKY DICK[3]

"In our age there is no such thing as 'keeping out of politics.' All issues are political issues, and politics itself is a mass of lies, evasions, folly, hatred and schizophrenia."

—GEORGE ORWELL
Futuristic Author of *1984* and *Animal Farm*

FROM A RECORDING of President Richard Nixon to H.R. "Bob" Haldeman, Oval Office, May 26, 1971, 10:03 a.m.:

---

[3] During his 1950 campaign for U.S. Senate, Richard Nixon was referred to as "Tricky Dick" by his opposition for alleged dirty campaign tactics (Gellman, Irwin (1999). *The Contender.* New York: The Free Press.)

NIXON: "Now, this is one thing I want. I want a goddam strong statement on marihuana. Can I get that out of this sonofabitching, uh, Domestic Council?"

HALDEMAN: "Sure."

NIXON: "I mean one on marihuana that just tears the ass out of them. I see another thing in the news summary this morning about it. You know it's a funny thing, every one of the bastards that are out for legalizing marihuana is Jewish. What the Christ is the matter with the Jews, Bob, what is the matter with them? I suppose it's because most of them are psychiatrists, you know, there's so many, all the greatest psychiatrists are Jewish. By God we are going to hit the marihuana thing and I want to hit it right square in the puss, I want to find a way of putting more on that . . ."

HALDEMAN: "Mm hmm, yep."

NIXON: I want to hit it, against legalizing and all that sort of thing."

PERHAPS RICHARD NIXON, like Harry Anslinger, had something to prove. His biographies certainly suggest as much. While the war on cannabis may have been waged effectively in 1937, Nixon revived it and expanded it in 1972. Instead of Mexicans and "darkies" to blame this time, it was homosexuals, Jews, and commies. That's despite the Nixon-appointed presidential commission that recommended cannabis be *neither* a state nor federal crime, and despite the opinions of close advisors to the same effect. Nixon simply over-ruled them, according to newly revealed declassified transcripts of recorded Oval Office conversations between 1971 and 1972.

In 1970 Congress passed the Controlled Substances Act which *temporarily* labeled cannabis a "Schedule I" substance—defined as an illegal drug which has no medical value. Congress at the same time admitted they knew too little about cannabis to make the designation permanent, so they created a presidential commission to look into cannabis and make recommendations for long-term policy. Nixon appointed anti-drug leaning members, including former Pennsylvania Governor Raymond Shafer. The National Commission on Marihuana and Drug Abuse or the "Shafer Commission" went about what would be the most comprehensive research project on cannabis ever performed by the Federal Government[4].

Despite the Commission's initial leanings, they began considering *legalization* of cannabis. Nixon had none of it, and months before the Commission was to issue its report, Nixon denounced them and their research, which led to a meeting between Shafer and Nixon. At that meeting Nixon demanded a strong anti-cannabis stance be taken by the Commission. Shafer assured Nixon he did not support legalization, although some members did. Nixon and Shafer also discussed the possibility of Shafer being appointed to a federal judgeship.

But the Commission didn't cave. Instead, it recommended a course to clear the "misinformation" surrounding cannabis, and tried to "demythologize" cannabis, and concluded cannabis did *not* cause an assortment of things previously accused of, such as:

- Leading to crime
- Leading to harder drug use
- Leading to aggression
- Causing abnormalities, whether physical or mental.

---

[4] With few exceptions, such as in rare federally-mandated cannabis research in the United States, the ability to research cannabis is almost completely precluded by its classification as a Schedule I substance. When we refer to research in this book and in the expansion of research, it is normally occurring *outside* the United States.

The commission stated:

> "Marihuana's relative potential for harm to the vast majority of individual users and its actual impact on society does not justify a social policy designed to seek out and firmly punish those who use it."

And they recommended *decriminalization* of "possession or non-profit transfer" of cannabis.

Nixon, again, had none of it. He proceeded on a course of "all-out war" on cannabis throughout the 1972 political season. He lumped cannabis among the other ills he sought to defeat, including, "homosexuality, dope, immorality in general." Within a year "marijuana" arrests jumped by over 30 percent, from 128,000 to 420,700. I guess when politics and prejudices were the priority, Nixon simply ignored the experts.

Today 650,000 people are arrested each year for possession of cannabis in the U.S. alone—750,000 arrests if you include other crimes such as dealing. And after almost a century of this costly "drug war" which might serve certain political expediencies, our prisons swell, and our society sinks deeper into drug-related crime and social problems. The rampant addiction today is not a cannabis problem, however, but rather a prescription-drug problem. Cannabis seems to have been forgotten or neglected in the mix, because it is still erroneously labeled a "Schedule 1" drug today. But that seems to be changing, and very quickly.

[3] BIG MEDICINE

"The truth is incontrovertible. Malice may attack it, ignorance may deride it, but in the end, there it is."
—WINSTON CHURCHILL
British Statesman, Orator, Author, and Prime Minister (1940–45, 1951–55)

IMAGINE THE FINANCIAL THREAT to Big Pharma posed by a "weed" (literally, that's how easy it grows) they can't control. They'd be about as excited as Big Oil if someone introduced a technology that allows cars to run on water. But most people just go along with full trust in the government and the FDA, and they don't do their own digging. Along the way they confirm those negative opinions of cannabis by the presence of "dope-smoking hippies," but the fact is Big Pharma has tentacles in medical schools and in the economics of research as well as health care, and people suffer needlessly as a result of these vested interests.

Medical schools today are *completely* subsidized by "Big Pharma," and it's not in Big Pharma's interests to have a side-effect free, all-natural *cure* for some of the things they treat *symptoms* of, at the great expense of patients. In medical school, you are supposed to learn the generic names of substances and use them in order to avoid bias. However, no one asks for a "facial tissue," they ask for a Kleenex. No one asks for "transparent tape," they ask for Scotch Tape—It's a matter of familiarity and branding. So, even as you're being trained to use the generic names of medications, the brand-names are catchier and easier to remember.

This guarantees that once students graduate they are most likely to use the brand-names. Large drug companies typically get involved in a medical school and the training of new doctors by the donation of equipment, books, and other things. When I was in training they used to come in and they would give us books or invite us to (or bring us) lunches or "educational" dinners, wherein they would promote their medications, of course. They would pay for a clinical trial or partner with the teaching institution in the clinical trials because that brings money to the institution as well as prestige.

From the 1900s and up into the 1950s and even the 1960s, there were medications that included cannabis. Big Pharma used cannabis as medicine. But in the early 1970s, our president at the time, Mr. Richard Nixon, had a daughter who was a big "pothead." As we've seen, like Harry Anslinger before him, Nixon spoke of the Hispanics and the blacks as dangerous "marijuana users," but Nixon also spoke of the "Jews" in that context as well. There are actual recordings and documents that prove all of this. We've seen some of the excerpts so far in this short book.

As a result of political incentives and economics, today the Board of Medicine and the Board of Osteopathic Medicine frown upon anything but what they deem "mainstream medicine," and that includes the use of cannabis, supplementation, bioidentical hormones, and even water because, again, there's no money in any of those for them. But doctors should learn natural remedies as well as synthetic ones. Cannabis is in the same boat as nutrition, supplements, and other natural remedies, and in fact, broadly neglected as a remedy.

As long as it is classed a "Schedule 1" illicit drug, no research can legally be done today (in the United States unless a specific exception is granted) into the efficacy and applications of cannabis as medicine, with few exceptions. In fact, "research" doesn't really exist in the United States today. The research that occurs here goes on because there's a financial gain to be made *by someone.* If I could do a clinical trial and prove that eating sugar—a certain candy bar, for example—cures cancer, I'm going to get support from where, do you suppose? The sugar industry, of course. So, it's based upon who is going to be able to make the greatest amount of cash. It's a horrible arrangement, and it's vast.

And it's not just cannabis. You might wonder why most doctors, when presented with your ailment, don't also at least include a prescription of *nutrition.* Most medical schools do not offer even one course in nutrition. We are always told, "Before you start any exercise program or supplementation, consult your doctor." It's done to prevent liability on the part of the supplier of the supplements.

When we're confronted with lies or major omissions, we have to first suspect there is something untrue or missing, and then with that verified, it helps to understand the "motive, means, and opportunity" behind the false or omitted information, and find out what the truth really is.

I can think of no subject where this is more important, relevant, and immediate, than when it comes to our health. In the next section, we'll (perhaps finally) make the nature of the cannabis plant clear and we'll see why it works so well, as far as we understand it today. But first, there may be a few last, additional road blocks to your "giving cannabis a chance," road blocks I run into all the time.

[4] STIGMAS

JUDGE: "Do the defendants have anything to say on their behalf before the court pronounces sentence?"

LEO BLOOM (played by Gene Wilder, stands up): "I would like to say something your honor, not on my behalf but in reference to my partner, Mr. Bialystock."

JUDGE: "Proceed."

LEO BLOOM: "Your honor, ladies and gentlemen of the jury, Max Bialystock is the most selfish man I ever met in my life."

MAX BIALYSTOCK (played by Zero Mostel): (tugs at Leo and whispers) "Don't help me!"

—*THE PRODUCERS* (1968)
Film by Mel Brooks

ON PERHAPS A lighter note, but no less serious if these are aspects that have slowed or stopped you from seeking the benefits to be had from medicinal cannabis, there are several social stigmas I'd like to address just briefly before we discuss the more serious aspects of the cannabis issue—what it takes to be a medical doctor who seeks all available and ideally natural remedies for their patients, how cannabis actually works in the human body, and what you do to become a properly supervised medical patient for whom cannabis is recommended.

In movies and pop culture, it's often joked about that in certain states where medical cannabis is legalized, people, with the cooperation of doctors, can obtain diagnoses such as "writer's cramp" and insomnia even if they don't actually suffer from these things in order to "get a med card" and be able to visit dispensaries (ones most notably that sell tobacco products) and buy the plant they will actually use for recreational purposes. For people only curious about the benefits of cannabis this can be a turn-off, and this representation is damaging to the cause of cannabis as true medicine. First, cannabis *is* an effective treatment for insomnia and maladies less severe than those terminal illnesses detailed in the current Florida law, and second, this makes the entire issue seem like a disguise for "pot heads" to legally obtain cannabis for recreation.

It's true, some will approach a physician in an attempt to secure legal, medicinal cannabis for recreational use, but we get these folks out of the office very quickly. We have a very strict screening process and *all* patients are well screened before they come in. In fact, there are a few simple safety protocols in place that make the process safe and secure and keep the product available for those who truly need it.

Another myth is that anyone open to cannabis use must certainly wear tie-dyes and go to pot festivals. It will be a cold day in hell before you catch me in a tie-dye, but I have to confess, I do actually have one. I have one particular suit which is off-white and 100-percent linen. I had three presentations one day and I was pretty exhausted. I had already done two, which were roundtables, and for the third, I was going to be on stage as the keynote speaker at an event. In between the two morning sessions and the afternoon session I was going by all of the display tables and ran into Chris Williams. He owns a company called "Sunshine Cannabis" and he has the market cornered on tie-dye shirts and hats. He saw me coming around, and I'm pretty well known in that arena, and he started screaming, "Dr. Rosado! Come here, come here!"

"What's going on, Chris?"

"That suit! I was going to wear a linen suit today but there's no way I was going to pull it off like you. I heard you were going to be wearing yours, so I have a shirt for you!"

"Alright," I said.

The color purple is the color for epilepsy awareness, and for that reason I had a white suit with a purple shirt. Chris gave me a purple tie-dye to wear, along with a white hat that has purple lettering on it, and he said, "When you're done on stage, after your talk, I want you to go behind the curtain, put the shirt and hat on and we'll snap a picture."

"Sure," I said. "I'll promote you that way, no problem." And that's the only time I've ever worn a tie-dye shirt. Another myth dispelled.

And contrary to what the Board of Medicine might say of "pot doctors," I didn't do this for money, either. It's accurate to say I am a pioneer in the field of medical marijuana. This is an *age* of medical cannabis pioneers, all across the United States. I have the scars to prove it, and I continue to fight, both in my professional as well as my personal life for this cause. Recreationally, cannabis is not my "drug of choice." Like most people, I tried it in high school. It did nothing for me, so I never participated. And that was it, recreationally, I was done.

All my work in this field is not just a front to get recreational marijuana legalized! In fact, because that's my position, because it's not a drug I use recreationally, many people *won't* come and see me. "How can I trust someone who doesn't participate?" they'll ask. But as in other fields of medicine, because I don't participate recreationally, it doesn't rule me out from seeing the medicinal attributes of cannabis and recommending it. There are doctors for example who, with their spouses, can't get pregnant and have children, but that doesn't preclude them from taking care of pregnant women.

I'm coming from the side of science. Yes, I'm an advocate, but I'm a physician first. Therefore, I am always going to be looking for the medical angle rather than the recreational angle. My involvement is purely medicinal. I have arrived where I am through a study of the facts. Ultimately, I came to the professional understandings I have of cannabis by way of medical journals and other facts. Early on, I was affiliated with friends and individuals who were moving in the direction of being advocates and recommending cannabis. Most of them, given the difficulties of occupying that space professionally, then decided to *not* go in that direction. Nonetheless they had a big impact on me. They left me intent on researching and learning more. The genie was out of the bottle.

Mainstream doctors are wary of recommending medical cannabis for various reasons—it's federally banned, for example, and there's little research on the drug's effectiveness for treating certain medical conditions (thanks mainly to the improper designation as having no medicinal value). They worry about liability and lawsuits. Because of that federal illegality, physicians' medical licenses could be at risk. In some cases, doctors are actually being discouraged by their hospital or other employer from talking to patients about the benefits of medical cannabis, much less recommending it. Yet we all take an oath to do no harm (and cannabis is virtually side-effect free), and my mandate as a physician is to help, however that might be accomplished.

Maybe discussing my professional difficulties will help engage us. I've been blocked by PayPal. Websites are often blocked if they discuss cannabis. We are not in the land of the free and the home of the brave. If you work for the state or you are at a government-sponsored facility such as a library, they are censoring the content you can access on their Wi-Fi, for example. Many doctors start down this road seeing the benefits and are deterred by the difficulties and bias and backlash and stigma they encounter along the way. It takes courage to be a "cannabis doctor," even though in so many cases it's the best, most beneficial treatment.

"I believe that a federal policy that prohibits physicians from alleviating suffering by prescribing marijuana for seriously ill patients is misguided, heavy-handed, and inhumane ... The government should change marijuana's status from that of a Schedule 1 drug (considered to be potentially addictive and with no current medical use) to that of a Schedule 2 drug (potentially addictive but with some accepted medical use) and regulate it accordingly."

—JEROME P. KASSIRER, MD
(Former) Editor, *New England Journal of Medicine*
"Federal Foolishness and Marijuana,"
Editorial of January 30, 1997

PART II: SCIENCE

[5] WHAT IS CANNABIS?

"Marijuana is no different than wine. It's a drug of choice. It's meant to alter your current state, and that's not a bad thing. It's ridiculous that marijuana is still illegal. We're still fighting for it."

—BRYAN CRANSTON
American Actor, Producer, Director, Screenwriter

S O, IF CANNABIS is *not* the downfall of humanity, *what is it?* It's a plant that occurs in nature, it's a weed. It certainly grows like one. But don't take my word for it. There is so much and so many clouding the issue, let's just stop for a minute and look at definitions:

"**A tall plant** with a stiff upright stem, divided serrated leaves, and glandular hairs. It is used to produce hemp fibre and as a drug." (emphasis added)

— OXFORD DICTIONARIES

"Cannabis is a genus of **flowering plants** in the family Cannabaceae." (emphasis added)

—WIKIPEDIA

"a **tall Asian herb** (Cannabis sativa of the family Cannabaceae, the hemp family) that has a tough fiber and is often separated into a tall loosely branched species (C. sativa) and a low-growing densely branched species (C. indica)" (emphasis added)

—MERRIAM-WEBSTER

". . . the word 'Cannabis' is not slang at all. Instead it is the accepted botanical Genus name for **the plant** we know by so many other slang and colloquial terms . . ." (emphasis added)

—URBANDICTIONARY.COM

So, it's a plant, a *weed* native to Asia and one that grows wild in lots of tropical areas across Earth. The flowering top (or simply the "flower") is cultivated and cured to use recreationally for the intoxicating effects, but in this book, we are talking about the *whole cannabis plant*, not just the flower, not just those parts of it that yield the highest concentrations of THC, unless of course the THC is what we are seeking for our *medicinal* purposes.

It has been made famous (or perhaps infamous) for its five-pronged, jagged leaves and distinctive odor, but it's basically a weed, it's a plant that occurs in nature. Most often, the flowers or "buds" and the leaves are used in medicine and recreationally, with the stalks and seeds used for myriad purposes (as we discuss next in the chapter on *hemp*). Typically, cannabis is smoked or eaten, or the extracted oil is ingested. We'll discuss preparations and what to expect from your doctor and your experience in this book as well. When a concentrated resin is extracted from cannabis and forms a sticky, often black liquid, this is called *hashish* or *hash oil*[5].

Regardless of form, all are products of the cannabis plant.

---

[5] "In the past, when a person wearing a leather dress moved between two rows of cannabis, at the end of these rows he would scrape off the resin stuck to the leather. The extract of this resin is usually called hash oil." —Professor Lumír Ondřej Hanuš

[6] WHAT IS HEMP?

"Some of my finest hours have been spent on my back veranda, smoking hemp and observing as far as my eye can see."

—THOMAS JEFFERSON
Founding Father of the United States

THERE IS OFTEN some confusion about cannabis and *hemp.* Hemp *is* cannabis. Basically, when we talk about cannabis in terms of a recreational drug, we are usually talking about the flower. When we talk about cannabis as a medicine, it might be the entire plant. When we talk about hemp, we are usually talking about the *same plant,* but in particular the stalks and seeds. According to Britannica.com, hemp is, "a tall cane-like variety" which is "raised for the production of hemp *fiber* (emphasis added), while the female plant of a short branchier variety is prized as the more abundant source of the psychoactive substance tetrahydrocannabinol (THC), the active ingredient of marijuana." Hemp *is* cannabis, and it does have THC, but normally not as much as cannabis cultivated for medicinal or recreational use.

Hemp has long been a cash crop for farmers because it grows quickly and in various conditions. Hemp *seed* is loaded with nutrition, and today we are using hemp to create useful products and even foods such as:

- Protein shakes and powder
- Milk
- Salad dressings
- Energy bars
- Fuel
- Biodegradable plastics

Hemp (cannabis) is apparently the earliest known woven fabric on this planet, going back 10,000 years, in addition to being used for medicine *just as long ago*. With so many varied uses, it's no surprise historians agree cannabis was the world's most cultivated plant for thousands of years. Prior to the more recent use of fossil fuels for plastics and other products, hemp was a fantastically popular material for making other valuables such as:

- Clothing, fiber, and fabric
- Paper
- Canvas
- Rope
- Lamp oil
- Medicine
- Incense

- Foods for people as well as animals (including porridge and soups from hemp seed)

In the south of France, they've discovered a bridge made from hemp hurds (the inner, woody part of the stalks) dating back to 600 A.D. Cannabis was an incredibly valuable crop for sailors, going back to early Viking explorers and European settlers. It's resistant to rot and salt, and so was used to make rigging and sails. It's said the USS Constitution was constructed with over *60 tons of hemp.* It was the "oil" of the past.

And since we've discussed the more recent laws that prohibit the use of cannabis, it's only balanced that we mention the previous laws *requiring* it. In the Jamestown Colony in 1619 a law was enacted that required *all* farmers to grow cannabis. More such laws were passed in Massachusetts in 1631, in Connecticut in 1632, and in the colonies in Chesapeake. Across the pond in England, it was decreed that foreigners who grew cannabis would be rewarded with full citizenship, and those who did not were often fined.

It was an important crop all over the world. Back in the Americas, from 1631 and up into the 19th century, you could even use cannabis as legal tender—part of encouraging the cultivation of it by farmers. George Washington and Thomas Jefferson grew it on their farms, and during those centuries you could even pay your taxes with it. In fact, Jefferson is said to have arranged for the illegal exportation of cannabis seeds from China to Turkey. China valued cannabis so much the exportation was a *capital offense.*

One of Benjamin Franklin's paper mills was started with locally-grown cannabis—a much better arrangement than getting their paper from England! All over the world most of the paper was made with hemp, right up until 1883. That included paper for newspapers, money, books, and bibles. Cannabis was also used to make fabrics (it's softer, stronger, and warmer than cotton) especially in Ireland and Italy. Even the most famous American flag, Old Glory, was made with cannabis fibers. In fact, the word *canvas* derives from *cannabis*. Right through the American Civil War most families had a "family hemp patch." Hemp rope was everywhere. In 1850 a U.S. census suggested there were over 8,000 hemp plantations, not including smaller, uncounted farms and family hemp patches. And it played a role in world affairs. Despite hemp being practically everywhere, the U.S. still couldn't get enough hemp and so imported it from Russia. To cut England's hemp supply line, Napoleon attacked Russia. The British, desperate for hemp, started attacking and capturing American ships.

And all over the world cannabis was a commonly used *medicine*, usually in the form of elixirs, tinctures, and extracts. It might have been the ibuprofen of the past, recommended for ailments such as:

- Depression and cramps from menstruation
- Migraine headaches
- Delirium tremens
- Asthma
- Rheumatism
- Cough
- Fatigue

So, what happened? The cotton gin, for one thing, making the use of cotton cheaper and easier. And as far as cannabis goes medically, the effects tended to vary from person to person as did the quality. In fact, we didn't "discover" THC until 1964 (THC was discovered in 1940 by Roger Adams, but its full and correct structure was only finally and fully understood in 1964 by Dr. Raphael Mechoulam.). And they certainly had none of the technology we now have for testing and cultivating cannabis. Next came the invention of the hypodermic needle, which made morphine the doctor's temporary drug of choice. The effects were fairly consistent, patient to patient, and the oil-based cannabis could not be injected. And to top it all off, we had the "reefer madness" propaganda campaign of the 1930s.

As discussed, the high probability is that vested interests could not tolerate a panacea that grows wild like a weed, with little or no side-effects, and this made cannabis a very big threat to certain pocketbooks.

[7] TYPES OF CANNABIS

"The anti-marijuana campaign is a cancerous tissue of lies, undermining law enforcement, aggravating the drug problem, depriving the sick of needed help and suckering well-intentioned conservatives and countless frightened parents."

—WILLIAM F. BUCKLEY JR.
American Editor, Author, and Intellectual Influence
in Conservative Politics

THERE ARE DIFFERENT TYPES of cannabis, and this can get confusing. Some subdivide cannabis into three subspecies (sativa, indica, ruderalis), some into two subspecies (sativa and indica, with ruderalis as a sub-category of sativa), and some refer to all cannabis as "sativa." For our purposes, and what seems to be the clearest way to understand the plant, is to divide cannabis into *two* categories because they have distinctly different effects when consumed or smoked:

- Sativa
- Indica

That said, many recreational forms of cannabis that are smoked are hybrids, or a cross between both types. With legalized cannabis and medical dispensaries, however, we have more control (and less worry) over cultivation and many strands have been now getting noticed for their outstanding medicinal results. For example, there are the (now famous) six Stanley brothers in Colorado who crossbred a strain of high-CBD, low-THC cannabis found to be effective in treating seizures in children, now called "Charlotte's Web," featured in a CNN special documentary titled, "Weed: A Dr. Sanjay Gupta Special." We'll discuss this incredible story later in the book.

That leaves us with *three basic types*: Cannabis Sativa, Cannabis Indica, and hybrids—much like wine is available in red, white, and blends of both. And regardless of what exotic label is attached to a particular chemovar (or subspecies), they all come from just those two subspecies: Cannabis Indica and Cannabis Sativa.

A basic familiarity with the two main types of cannabis will make obvious some of the potential medicinal applications:

Sativa
- High THC level
- Best suited for day use
- Energetic and uplifting
- Spacey, cerebral, or hallucinogenic

- Stimulates appetite
- Relieves depression
- Slender leaf shape
- Grows tall, up to 20 feet
- Flavor is typically earthy

Indica
- High CBD level
- Best suited for night use
- Calming, sedating, and relaxing
- "Couch lock" or body buzz
- Stimulates appetite
- Reduces anxiety and pain
- Wide leaf shape
- Grows 3-4 feet typically
- Flavor is typically sweet

[8] HOW DOES IT WORK?

"Prohibition… goes beyond the bounds of reason in that it attempts to control mans' appetite through legislation and makes a crime out of things that are not even crimes… A prohibition law strikes a blow at the very principles upon which our Government was founded."

—ABRAHAM LINCOLN

16th president of the United States from 1861 until his assassination in April 1865

THROUGH THE AGES we have discovered cannabis has medicinal properties. In fact, cannabis was introduced to the United States as a *medicinal* product in the mid-1800s and was widely recommended by physicians for various ailments until 1937, when, as discussed, penalties were created to prevent its medical or recreational use with the Marijuana Tax Act. Prohibition culminated in 1970 with the passage of the Controlled Substance Act, which formalized the criminalization of marijuana possession or use, regardless of quantity or context. Yet, despite its "illegal" status, public demand for medical access led to the legalization of cannabis for medical use in California in 1996, and as of 2018, voters in an additional 33 states, the District of Columbia, Puerto Rico, and Guam have followed suit. Not all of these voters are recreational users. Cannabis is gaining legal acceptance in tidal-wave-like fashion across the United States (and the world) because *it works*.

Despite the long history of cannabis as a natural plant with medicinal benefits, our understanding of how it works in the human body at a cellular level has only recently become clearer. In the 1960s a scientist in Israel named Raphael Mechoulam[6] is often credited with discovering what we now know as THC, or *tetrahydrocannabinol*[7]. This is the main psychoactive

---

[6] Raphael Mechoulam's major scientific interest is the chemistry and pharmacology of cannabinoids. He and his research group succeeded in the total synthesis of the major plant cannabinoids Δ9-tetrahydrocannabinol, cannabidiol, cannabigerol and various others. Another research project initiated by him led to the isolation of the first described endocannabinoid anandamide which was isolated and characterized by two of his postdoctoral researchers, Lumír Ondřej Hanuš and William Devane. Another endogenous cannabinoid, 2-AG, was soon discovered by Shimon Ben-Shabat, one of his PhD students. He published more than 350 scientific articles. — Michael Denman (2007), "MECHOULAM, RAPHAEL", Encyclopaedia Judaica, 13 (2nd ed.), Thomson Gale, pp. 711–712

[7] "With all my respect to professor Mechoulam, in 1964 Yehiel Gaoni and Raphael Mechoulam in Israel isolated THC and elucidated its structure. In the same year, František Šantavý in Czechoslovakia elucidated not only the structure of THC but also its absolute configuration. THC, however, had already been isolated and named in 1940 by Roger Adams, who suggested its structure but there was just one

agent found in the cannabis plant. It's what produces the "high" people feel when smoking or ingesting cannabis. That was just the beginning of our understanding of how cannabis works and why it seems to work so well with the human body. THC was isolated and tested as to its medicinal benefits against many other cannabinoids found in the plant, but it would be another several decades before we made any large advances in that knowledge.

In the 1980s, the receptor in the human brain that works with THC was discovered and dubbed *cannabinoid receptor 1* or "CB1." But why was there a receptor naturally existing in the *human brain* for THC? Did it receive other signals as well? Researchers expanded their investigation to include not only cannabinoids found in the cannabis plant, but also for potentially naturally occurring cannabinoids in the human body, *and they found them!* These, because they are naturally produced by the human body (or "endogenous," or "occurring from within") were called *endocannabinoids.*

The first endocannabinoid, the first such compound that was found to naturally occur in the human body, was a neurotransmitter they called *anandamide.* It was also called the "bliss compound," as it was found to stimulate feelings of joy and happiness. Chemically, anandamide is different than THC, but like THC, it binds to the CB1 receptor and stimulates the exact same effects as THC does—*happiness.*

Then a second brain receptor was discovered, albeit in lesser quantity than CB1, called CB2 (of course). This new (to us) receptor has a close relationship to the human immune system, as it was mainly found in high concentrations in various parts of the body, all related to immune function. And today, we are aware of many natural compounds that act upon or bind with these two

mistake—the position of the double bond in the terpenic cycle." — Professor Lumír Ondřej Hanuš receptors, CB1 and CB2, such as *cannabidiol,* or CBD, for example. CBD oil is legal and used for medicinal purposes all over the United States today, and is a natural compound found in the cannabis plant. Such substances are called *cannabinoids.* Compounds produced naturally within the human body (called *endocannabinoids*) include:

- Anandamide (AEA)
- 2-Arachidonoylglycerol (2-AG)
- And many more

As far as we now know, CB1 and CB2 are the two primary components of the human *endocannabinoid system.* And there are today known to be 144 phytocannabinoids[8] within the cannabis plant, yet to be fully researched and fully understood. They are all of potentially great health, medicinal, and curative value. Yet, *research* is still illegal in many places (at least in the United States), and the ability to research is just one of the many arguments for legalization of medical cannabis. It is presumed that there are many more receptors and many more endocannabinoids yet to be found by current and future research.

And yes, you read that right, there exists a *human endocannabinoid system,* akin to other systems found in the human body (such as the endocrine system, nervous system, lymphatic system, and so on). It's quite a discovery. *Endocannabinoids* are found throughout the human body—in fact they are found throughout the bodies of *all* other vertebrate animals and even throughout the bodies of certain invertebrate animals.

Remember, *endogenous cannabinoids* are the chemicals our own bodies make to naturally stimulate the

---

[8] **Phytocannabinoids**: cannabinoids that occur naturally in the cannabis plant — https://www.news-medical.net/

human cannabinoid receptors, CB1 and CB2. And as mentioned, the two most well-known endogenous cannabinoids (or endocannabinoids) are again, anandamide and 2-arachidonoylglycerol (2-AG). It may be worth adding that CB1 receptors are mainly found in the human brain and human reproductive organs, and CB2 receptors are found throughout the human peripheral nervous system (PNS) as well as throughout the human immune system.

Some people need THC because of what's called the entourage effect, where the CBD together with the THC works synergistically in the different receptors in the brain, spinal cord, and peripheral nervous system. The THC component is needed because their issue may be not so much in the peripheral nervous system, but more in the central nervous system, where THC works.

It's as if this was all planned by nature!

You don't necessarily have to remember all of these technical aspects. The point is simply that these things have been found to be naturally present and work a certain way in the human body—we are not introducing anything synthetic when we deal with all-natural cannabis, unlike many pharmaceuticals today. In fact, activities such as exercise support the endogenous production of cannabinoids. We might all be familiar with "runner's high"? Well, the human body produces these endocannabinoids in a similar fashion to how it produces endorphins.

And further, the endocannabinoid system alters CB1 or CB2 receptor expressions during stress response, which is beneficial in some pathologic states (such as neuropathic pain and multiple sclerosis), because increased CB expression may lessen symptoms or disease progression and provide a protective role as well.

Most cannabinoids (again, the natural compounds within the cannabis plant) will not get you high. THC is the only one known to do that with certainty. And you won't get high just by eating raw cannabis. In fact, cannabis does *not* directly produce either THC or CBD, the two substances most consumers are looking for. But when you heat cannabis sufficiently, you activate the acids found in the plant and that is what yields the THC and the CBD. This is why people either smoke cannabis or eat or ingest it after it has been cooked or extracted in some form.

And while THC is famous for its intoxicating effects, other cannabinoids have other effects when activated or heated, like insecticidal or antibiotic effects. It's believed these effects are a way nature designed for the plant to defend itself under certain circumstances. And heat seems to change the acidic nature of a substance like THCA into a non-acidic form with (simply) THC.

This is found elsewhere in nature, of course. Fires and controlled burns are used to clear and regenerate forests by removing the dead and decayed material and clear the way for new growth. The jack pine, for example, has resin-filled cones that must be melted by fire before they burst open and release seeds. And as most of us probably experience each day in some fashion, it's *roasting* that changes green coffee beans into dark brown ones and triggers the chemical reactions within the coffee that produces the flavors we all seem to love so much. It's the fire and heat that enact the actual chemical and physical transformations of the coffee bean into something we buy at coffee shops.

Cannabis, like every other plant on Earth, has within it essential oils called *terpenes.* The terpenes provide unique smells and flavors, as well as the unique *feeling* each cannabis plant provides. In fact, two cannabis plants of similar strains and of similar structure can have vastly different effects, depending on the terpenes. In *sativa* strains, the aroma is typically bright and often like citrus— in fact the type of terpene that supplies this flavor is called *limonene,* and is the same terpene found in lemons. Limonene, in addition to the citrus flavor it provides, also supplies an uplifting feeling, stimulates the immune system, and provides defense for your GI tract.

Indica strains of cannabis on the other hand smell more like pine trees—in fact these terpenes, *alpha and beta pinene*, are the same as found in pine trees. Pinene also provides relief from pain thanks to its anti-inflammatory properties. Another terpene found in indica strains of cannabis is often *linalool,* a floral-smelling substance also found in lavender.

Terpenes affect us when they are smelled and inhaled. We get a small sampling of the cannabis this way. And this "sampling" can give an early indication of how each particular cannabis strain will affect us, and how each will interact with our own body chemistry. *The appeal or lack of it the smell or flavor of each cannabis strain has for you is indeed a good indication of how much you will like or not like each strain and can be as large a factor in the effects as the THC level of each plant.*

So exactly like becoming a connoisseur of wine, cigars, flowers, food, or chocolate, it's okay and even encouraged to sniff, evaluate, note your responses and use words like "oaky, floral, piney, citrusy, woody," and "hints of lavender." And also to note your reactions such as "stimulated" or "soothing." And if you really enjoy this aspect and might enjoy becoming a true aficionado, there are whole charts created (on the website Leafly, for example) that look like color wheels, noting the types of terpenes and their effects.

[9] BENEFITS OF CANNABINOIDS

"The illegality of cannabis is outrageous, an impediment to full utilization of a drug which helps produce the serenity and insight, sensitivity and fellowship so desperately needed in this increasingly mad and dangerous world."

—CARL SAGAN
Astronomer and Astrophysicist

CANNABINOIDS, THE NATURAL compounds found in the cannabis plant, continue to reveal to us various and abundant health benefits as we continue to research. The THC found in cannabis is more of a stimulant than CBD and has the following benefits:

- Reduces pain
- Kills malignant cells (apoptosis)
- Reduces the vomiting and exhaustion as a result of chemotherapy and radiation treatment
- Stimulates appetite
- Relieves symptoms that accompany asthma and bronchitis
- Reduces or eliminates various seizures
- Supports circadian rhythm and reverses sleep disorders and insomnia
- Relieves those suffering from PTSD and other stress
- Acts as a general antidepressant

The CBD found in cannabis and hemp is more sedative in nature, and has the following benefits:

- Is not psychoactive
- Is a potent antioxidant
- Reduces anxiety, agitation, and panic attacks
- Creates a relaxed and stable frame of mind
- Offers many anti-cancer benefits

The CBN found in cannabis offers the following benefits that we are now aware of:

- Pain relief
- Anti-epilepsy benefits
- Lowers the buildup of pressure in the eyes

Other cannabinoids such as CBC (cannabichromene) both support and consolidate the effects of THC. The cannabinoid CBG (cannabigerol) is an effective anti-inflammatory agent with calming, sedative-like properties.

These are only some of the known benefits of cannabinoids, and perhaps even more importantly, only some of the cannabinoids we are aware of through research. We now know of at least 144 phytocannabinoids in the cannabis plant, and these above are just a few that occur naturally (in the cannabis plant).

While these individual cannabinoids have great benefits, the greatest benefit is arguably what they all do *together*. It's called the "entourage effect" and it describes how these compounds work most effectively when together, synergistically. Many compounds in cannabis seem at first to do very little on their own, but when working in unison with other cannabinoids, enhance the effects of others. This is important because drug companies are starting to produce "synthetic cannabis," despite the fact that we are not yet even aware of all cannabinoids and what they do. Another reason natural is better.

These benefits are just a start. Listed below are some of the known cannabinoid compounds and their associated disorders they have been shown to help with. We'll break them down into five general categories of benefit, then list the cannabinoids, then the conditions those cannabinoids help with. As you'll see, there are many, and much more to learn about these and other cannabinoids that occur naturally in the cannabis plant:

1. Pain/Sleep
   - THC
     - Sleep Apnea
   - CBD, THC
     - Cramps
     - Migraine/Headache
     - Phantom Limb
     - Spinal Injury
   - CBD, CBN, THC

- Fibromyalgia
  - CBC, CBD, CBN, THC
    - Insomnia
  - CBC, CBD, CBN, THC, THCv
    - Pain
  - CBC, CBD, CBDa, CBG, CBN, THC, THCa
    - Arthritis
    - Inflammation

2. Gastro-Intestinal
   - THC
     - Appetite Loss
   - CBD, THC
     - Anorexia
     - Cachexia
     - Gastrointestinal Disorders
     - Nausea
   - CBD, THCv
     - Diabetes
   - CBD, THC, THCa
     - Crohn's

3. Mood/Behavior
   - CBD, CBG
     - Anxiety
   - CBD, THC
     - ADD/ADHD
     - Stress
   - CBD, CBG, THC
     - Bipolar
     - OCD
     - PTSD
   - CBC, CBD, CBG, CBN, THC
     - Depression

4. Neurological
   - THC
     - Tourette's
   - CBD, CBN, THCa, THCv
     - Epilepsy
     - Seizures
   - CBC, CBN, THC, THCa
     - Multiple Sclerosis
   - CBC, CBD, CBG, THC, THCa
     - Alzheimer's
     - Parkinson's
   - CBD, CBG, CBN, THC, THCa
     - Spasticity
   - CBC, CBD, CBG, CBN, THCv
     - Osteoporosis
   - CBC, CBD, CBG, CBN, THC, ThCa
     - ALS

5. Other
   - THC
     - Fatigue
     - Asthma
   - CBD, THC
     - Hypertension
   - CBG, THC
     - Glaucoma
   - THC, THCa
     - HIV/AIDS
   - CBC, CBD, CBG, THC
     - Muscular Dystrophy
   - CBC, CBD, CBDa, CBG, THC, THCa
     - Cancer

One of the established health benefits of cannabis and endocannabinoids is the contribution they make to *homeostasis,* or the state of health wherein the various parts of the human body are harmoniously working together in a sort of balance. This means better dealing with stress, fighting off disease, and faster healing. It relates to our ability to defend against toxicity and poor diet as well as against the high levels of stress in the civilization today. We have also discovered the endocannabinoid system can be damaged and left deficient, but that it can be repaired by supplementing with the phytocannabinoids found in the cannabis plant.

Are you starting to see why Big Pharma might not like the idea of all of these things being nicely handled by a plant that grows like a weed? The natural compounds in cannabis perfectly mimic the natural compounds the human body produces which are so vital for the endocannabinoid system and homeostasis. This makes "whole plant" therapy important as we are not completely aware of or able to replicate *all* of the synergistic compounds in cannabis. It explains why cannabis is so beneficial for our health, so easy to administer, and so free of side-effects. Perhaps it explains why so many vested interests fight its release and legalization so fervently, as well.

When you consider the side-effects of so many pharmaceuticals, when you hear them whispered rapidly throughout a television commercial (over images of smiling, happy people), it can make you feel you've stepped into a horror film of sorts. Pharmaceutical companies are required to disclose known side-effects. They can be horrible—often as or more horrible than the malady they are designed to "treat," and these side-effects comprise the pages of tomes such as *Meyler's Side-effects of Drugs: The International Encyclopedia of Adverse Drug Reactions and Interactions.*

Yet in my experience as a physician, the administration of medicinal cannabis leads either to very mild side-effects or, usually, none at all. A side effect known as "greening out" can be quite common in people who have not used cannabis or have used non-medical grade cannabis. The following are the symptoms of too much marijuana in the system:

- Temporary feelings of paranoia, fear and anxiety
- Shortness of breath
- Pupil dilation
- Vomiting and/or nausea
- Fast heart rate
- Shaking that is hard to control, feeling cold
- Disorientation or hallucinations
- Hangover

This phenomenon passes on its own within minutes to hours of marijuana use and is part of the argument for professionally-administered type and dosage of medical cannabis according to a trained physician's recommendations.

Of course, results aren't typical for everyone. And it is possible, especially in combination with other risk factors, that one might form a psychological addiction with anything so palliative as cannabis and turn to substance abuse. But this has not been my experience with *medically recommended* cannabis, and when weighed against the inefficacy and drawbacks of other alternatives, treatment with cannabis stands out as vastly preferable.

What does all of this mean? It means if you are honest about the facts, cannabis helps. It means the human body has the infrastructure in place to make use of the compounds found in cannabis for better health and improved mental state. We were apparently *designed* that way. It's at least a little amazing that the compounds in cannabis (phytocannabinoids) are so similar to others naturally produced, found, and used in the human body (endocannabinoids), and that these bioidentical compounds are all very readily used by our bodies for improvement and health and with virtually no side-effects.

"Estimates suggest that from 20 to 50 million Americans routinely, albeit illegally, smoke marijuana without the benefit of direct medical supervision. Yet, despite this long history of use and the extraordinarily high numbers of social smokers, there are simply no credible reports to suggest that consuming marijuana has caused a single death. By contrast, aspirin, a commonly used, over-the-counter medicine, causes hundreds of deaths each year."

—FRANCIS YOUNG
Former DEA Chief Administrative Law Judge

PART III: LAW

[10] APPROVED DIAGNOSES

"I'm going to look at starting a fund where we all can donate to get full marijuana legalization on the ballot in 2020. When you mess with the will of the people there are unintended consequences! The cannabis industry is well funded now. Money won't be a problem. #ForThePeople"

—JOHN MORGAN
Founder, Morgan & Morgan
On Twitter, June 26, 2018

ONE WAY TO NAVIGATE these tricky waters as a doctor is to be vigilant and to know and follow the current laws *to the letter*. If you engage in this type of practice as a physician, you cannot have a bank account in a regular bank. Remember, federally, it's illegal and the FDIC will come down on you. You can't then, use credit cards, or make "normal" deposits. You have to use a bank that is cannabis-friendly. And they exist. They're called "green banks," and in Florida, there actually is now a bank called "Green Bank." At this writing they are the only bank that does accept and service cannabis-friendly medical practitioners.

But again, there is a way to safely accomplish this, a way to participate and benefit from cannabis as a patient, and that way is *carefully.* Find licensed, professional, careful, knowledgeable medical practitioners. If you're local, come in and consult with me. If you have questions about symptoms, contact my office. There is a way to do everything above board, and that includes finding and connecting with those professionals like myself, who are as careful and informed as we need to be.

I have patients who come in from all parts of Florida. I'm an early adopter, I'm factually a pioneer. I was one of the first in the State of Florida to get certified. I was the first to professionally recommend cannabis in the Greater Central Florida area (Volusia, Orange, Seminole, Osceola counties). The years that I've dedicated to learning about this and the trade, not only the medical side of things but also the business, financial, horticultural, and legal side of things, inform me that it's more than just writing a recommendation and having a line up to my front door. We need to stop throwing out the baby with the bathwater, but we do need to throw away the dirty bath water! May the stigmas and difficulties go with it.

For many years, the people of Florida have been getting louder and more numerous when it comes to demanding access to medical cannabis. This resulted in action in 2014, and steady progress for legalization ever since. In fact, often what slows a state down in approving medical cannabis is not a moral or ethical mater but a *legal* one, as states watch to see what other states go through in the process of legalization.

Florida *started* legalization of cannabis in 2014, but in a very limited yet worthy way. With the passage of Senate Bill 1030 (SB1030), which then-Governor Rick Scott signed into law on June 16th, 2014, low-level THC-cannabis-only was approved, and only for children. It was called the "Charlotte's Web Bill" in reference to the surprising and course-altering appearance of a low-grade strain of cannabis that helped a little girl overcome her daily seizures in Colorado when nothing else seemed to work for her. The passage of SB1030 meant to many in Florida that kids suffering from seizures and other conditions would now be able to live more normal lives with less suffering.

Senate Bill 1030:

- Defined "medical use"
- Created the Compassionate Care Registry (the official list of those in Florida qualified as dispensing organizations and those qualified as patients—children only at the time)
- Required doctors to submit quarterly reports to the University of Florida School of Pharmacy to study the effectiveness of treatments
- Divided Florida into five sections, each with a legally observed dispensary to serve it
- Determined that state research funds should be used to study the effectiveness of medical cannabis
- And required a doctor's recommendation of medical cannabis be supported by the signature of a second qualified physician

What Senate Bill 1030 really did, even more basically than allowing low-grade cannabis for certain children, was create a needed framework *and set an important precedent* for future expansion of medical cannabis (and possibly even recreational) in the State of Florida. A vote on "Amendment 2" was to take place in the near future.

Two years later, the people of Florida approved the Florida Medical Marijuana Legalization Initiative, also called "Amendment 2," on November 8th, 2016, approving the use of cannabis for medical purposes in the alleviation of debilitating medical conditions. It was approved by 6,518,919 votes *yes* (71%) and 2,621,845 voting *no* (28%), according to the Florida Secretary of State. The goal of the bill was to help alleviate the suffering of anyone in the State of Florida with a debilitating condition. It's from Amendment 2 that we get our list of diagnoses for which medical cannabis can be recommended (listed later in this chapter and discussed in more detail in the next section).

With Amendment 2 medical cannabis could now be recommended by a qualified physician if they believed the benefits of use outweigh the potential health risks. It allowed, specifically, the use of medical cannabis by taking pills, sprays, oils, or vaping, but prohibited the smoking of cannabis (which only now has become allowed by Florida law at this writing).

The Florida Department of Health has created a nice infographic that explains the timeline of implementation of the law allowing medical cannabis in Florida, summarized here for your interest:

FLORIDA DEPARTMENT OF HEALTH
Office of Compassionate Use
Low-THC Cannabis & Medical Cannabis
Implementation Timeline

- July 1, 2014: Office of Compassionate Use Established

- May 28, 2015: Florida Administrative Code Chapter 64-4 Final Rule Upheld. Effective on June 17, 2015

- July 8, 2015: Dispensing Organization Applications Accepted

- Nov. 23, 2015: Dispensing Organizations Announced
  1. CHT Medical
  2. Knox Medical
  3. Modern Health Concepts
  4. Surterra Therapeutics
  5. Trulieve

- Dec. 14, 2015: Challenges Received: 13 Administrative Petitions and 1 Counter Petition

- Feb. 5, 2016: Five Dispensing Organizations Request Cultivation Authorization / Dispensing Organizations Granted Cultivation Authorization:

  o Surterra Therapeutics (Feb. 17, 2016)
  o Trulieve (Feb. 29, 2016)
  o Modern Health Concepts (Mar. 14, 2016)
  o CHT Medical (June 22, 2016)
  o Knox Medical (July 7, 2016)

- Mar. 25, 2016: Governor Scott signs HB 307 into Law

- Apr. 6, 2016: The Green Solution (San Felasco Nursery) Approved as sixth dispensing organization

- July 11, 2016: Compassionate Use Registry Available

- July 12, 2016: All Dispensing Organizations Cultivating Cannabis

- July 22, 2016: Dispensing Began in Florida

At this writing, the current law regulating the recommendation by physicians and use by patients of cannabis in Florida is Senate Bill 8A ("SB 8-A Medical Use of Marijuana"), the official summary of which states:

> Medical Use of Marijuana; Providing an exemption from the state tax on sales, use, and other transactions for marijuana and marijuana delivery devices used for medical purposes; providing qualifying medical conditions for a patient to be eligible to receive marijuana or a marijuana delivery device; providing for the establishment of medical marijuana testing laboratories; establishing the Coalition for Medical Marijuana Research and Education within the H. Lee Moffitt Cancer Center and Research Institute, Inc., etc. APPROPRIATION: $15,143,440.00
> Effective Date: 6/23/2017

To be able to recommend medical cannabis in the state of Florida, a licensed physician must take an 8-hour course and pass the subsequent exam. There are diagnoses that are specifically named and allowed for cannabis recommendations in the current Florida law, and many people assume these are the only conditions for which cannabis can currently be recommended but that is not true. There is a provision in current Florida law that states any certified physician who deems the use of cannabis more beneficial than detrimental for a patient can prescribe cannabis for that patient, even outside of the diagnoses specifically mentioned. You have to fill out a document and submit it to the State of Florida. You have to provide supporting documentation that equates that condition with one of the existing conditions, but it is provided for in the current law.

Those diagnoses named and for which the State of Florida will legally allow the recommendation of cannabis as treatment by licensed, regulated physicians are listed below:

1. Cancer
2. Epilepsy
3. Glaucoma
4. HIV
5. AIDS
6. PTSD (Post-Traumatic Stress Disorder)
7. ALS (Amyotrophic Lateral Sclerosis)
8. Crohn's disease
9. Parkinson's disease
10. MS (Multiple Sclerosis)

Conditions comparable to those above include chronic, nonmalignant pain caused by or originating or persisting from a condition listed above, other terminal conditions, and more.

And while that's *what's* covered, there are three classes of people *who* are covered:

1. **Qualified patients**: "A person who has been added to the Medical Marijuana Use Registry by a qualified physician and can buy medical marijuana and devices using their ID card."

2. **Caregiver**: "A person who has agreed to assist a qualified patient and has a caregiver ID card."

3. **Qualified physician**: "A physician who is certified to order low-THC cannabis, medical marijuana and delivery devices for a qualified patient, and is in the Medical Marijuana Use Registry."

It's my hope in this book to demystify and give a more professional aspect to the field I love, so that people all over the state who suffer any of these diagnoses will feel empowered to seek the best possible solutions available to them and their loved ones. Things *are changing*. Legalization of cannabis in tobacco form is currently under discussion (among *eleven* current lawsuits against the state) and a new (federally chartered) bank has already said it will come to Florida:

> "Foreseeing 'a multibillion-dollar industry here,' the head of Seattle-based GRN Funds says his firm has come to Florida to offer banking services to the state's medical marijuana providers."

This will mean more physicians will be able and willing to recommend cannabis for its healing properties, and rather than being misunderstood due to antiquated propaganda, cannabis can take its rightful place as an all-natural, side-effect-free solution, highly regarded and understood for its many benefits, researched, recommended, and openly discussed in the light of day.

In the meantime, we can and do now have stated goals for treatment when employing medical cannabis in the case of these various diagnoses.

- Cancer: Manage nausea, vomiting, anorexia, weight loss, restore the immune system, etc.

- Epilepsy: Decrease the number of seizures per day, week, or month and wean off of the multiple AEDs (antiepileptic drugs).

- Glaucoma: Decrease the intraocular pressure.

- HIV (human immunodeficiency virus) and AIDS (acquired immune deficiency syndrome): Manage the wasting syndrome and restore the immune system.

- PTSD (post-traumatic stress disorder): Address the anxiety, depression, night terrors, etc.

- ALS (amyotrophic lateral sclerosis, abnormal hardening of body tissue): Manage the muscle spasms and pain associated with the spasms.

- Crohn's disease: Manage the GI (gastrointestinal) symptoms and address the anorexia, weight-loss, and restore the immune system.

- Parkinson's disease: Decrease and/or eliminate the resting tremors, bradykinesia[9] and dyskinesia (impairment of voluntary movement).

- MS (multiple sclerosis): Manage the muscle spasms and pain associated with the spasms.

Doctors are now getting more experience with the recommending of medical cannabis and researchers are discovering more about its prescription and use as the legal binds are loosened across the United States and all over the world. It's a doctor's job to heal, and first, to do no harm. When we look at what medical cannabis can do and what it might potentially do as we better understand and use it, both of these standards can be more easily achieved with patients.

---

[9] Bradykinesia means slowness of movement and is one of the cardinal manifestations of Parkinson's disease. Weakness, tremor and rigidity may contribute to but do not fully explain bradykinesia. — https://academic.oup.com/brain/article/124/11/2131/302768

[11] BECOMING A PATIENT

"If you substitute marijuana for tobacco and alcohol, you'll add eight to 24 years to your life."

—JACK HERER
American Cannabis Rights Activist and Author

HOW DO YOU become a patient who is recommended medical cannabis in the State of Florida? The first step in becoming a legal medical cannabis patient is seeing a qualified physician for a certification exam. According to SB1030, passed in 2014, to be a Florida cannabis patient, you must be "suffering from cancer or a physical medical condition that chronically produces symptoms of seizures or severe and persistent muscle spasms" and your qualified physician may then recommend for your medical use low-THC cannabis to alleviate your symptoms, if no other satisfactory alternative treatment options exist for you. Additionally, you must be a permanent resident of Florida, and have established a 90-day doctor-patient relationship.

When Amendment 2 was passed in 2016, it was further defined that to be a medical cannabis patient you must have a debilitating condition such as: "cancer, epilepsy, glaucoma, positive status for human immunodeficiency virus (HIV), acquired immune deficiency syndrome (AIDS), post- traumatic stress disorder (PTSD), amyotrophic lateral sclerosis (ALS), Crohn's disease, Parkinson's disease, multiple sclerosis, or other debilitating medical conditions of the same kind or class as or comparable to those enumerated, and for which a physician believes that the medical use of marijuana would likely outweigh the potential health risks for a patient."

And now, "as of March 2017, all patients and legal representatives must obtain a Registry Identification Card to fill an order for low-THC cannabis, medical cannabis, or a cannabis delivery device at one of the state's dispensing organizations." To apply to become a patient and obtain a registry identification card, you must be a Florida resident, suffer from a qualifying, debilitating condition, and submit a completed application to the Florida Office of Medical Marijuana Use.

To get your online application process started, you first have your qualifying physician enter your email address into the online registry. You are then immediately sent an email that allows you to start the process for obtaining your medical marijuana card in Florida. Currently, your photo is uploaded from the department of motor vehicles, and you'll need a registration fee of $75. Cards remain active for one year. You may get a temporary card until your permanent card arrives in the form of an e-mail from the Office of Medical Marijuana Use, which allows you to go to any dispensary in the state of Florida and purchase your medicine.

As you can see, the way you go about getting cannabis recommended and administered is different than a typical written script from your doctor. It's much more precise and more carefully monitored than that. As just mentioned, your cannabis-indoctrinated physician first enters your recommendation into a digital statewide patient registry. There's no writing of a paper prescription, per se. I, or your qualified physician, put in the order or the recommendation online. You then go to one of the various dispensaries across the state of Florida. The dispensary administrator looks you up and sees the order I've entered for you. The dispensary then tells you (the patient) what you are able to obtain, based on my recommendation. You then choose from available and recommended products from a menu.

I, as your physician, enter what I recommend as your recommended dosage, and I then also guide you through your available choices as far as administering your cannabis. Available products have included oils and as of March 2019, Florida Governor Ron DeSantis signed into law SB 182, allowing the smokable version of medical cannabis. If you do vaping, one three-second inhalation yields 1.6 milligrams of THC. If you are doing sublingual or oral oil, then the dropper has a gauge on there (0.25, 0.5, 0.75, or 1 milliliter), or you can get a syringe and you are supplied with a sheet that explains, for example, 0.1 milliliter yields so many milligrams of THC. So, if I've recommended, say, 5 milligrams, your sheet will guide you through how much oil to take with the dropper to reach your dosage of 5 milligrams. There are nasal sprays, metered dose inhalers, dry flower vape cups, capsules, oral sprays, topical creams, patches, and suppositories. Although edibles are allowed per SB 8A, at the writing of this book, the Florida Department of Health has yet to have provided direction to the Medical Marijuana Treatment Centers on how to go about dispensing edibles.

You get instruction from me (your primary care doctor will likely have no clue as to how to go about this) and from the state-approved dispensary. And what I've just described for purposes of example, are how things are currently done in the State of Florida. In other states it can be completely different. It's an efficient process for the most part and easy to follow, nothing mysterious about it, all tightly regulated and intended for those with the lawful state-specified diagnoses or other instances where I decide the benefit of cannabis would outweigh any drawbacks for your particular case. It's all carefully done, and a digital accounting of everything is created. I also have you keep a log or a journal of how you are doing. That way when you come in I can evaluate and decide based on results what in your case needs to be done.

There are now available (in Florida) products that are low-THC and products that are high-THC—the psychoactive agent in cannabis. There will be a sense of euphoria when taking products that include high-THC. CBD products are low-THC. Both are available in the state of Florida. What I recommend for you is case-specific and all depends on what is appropriate for you and your situation, based on your diagnosis.

Some of these products have become very well known. A product we have mentioned, a strain called "Charlotte's Web" is a low-THC product famous for alleviating seizures in young children, and which has, due to availability, prompted a migration of many families to Colorado, where they can easily and legally obtain it for their children. Hailey's Hope is another low-THC product, as are Palmetto Harmony, Mindful Medicinals, and Green Roads World. These are all low-THC and available over the counter, which you can buy without a recommendation. They each come from hemp, and hemp is legal in all 50 states, according to the Farm Bill of 2018. Sanjay Gupta did a fantastic documentary on this for CNN, which I recommend.

Originally there were five "holders" or state-approved cannabis growers in Florida, but by now there are growers all over Florida, growing the medication for all of the dispensaries. That number keeps growing, and while there are between 11 to 14 licensed holders I'm aware of at this writing, there may be more already. And while these I've mentioned are all licensed holders, they are not all dispensing. They are in different phases of the process. There are currently just a handful who are both growing and dispensing, and they are in South Florida, Central Florida, and Northwest Florida. There are "grows" outside of Tampa, outside of Tallahassee, Lake Worth, and more popping up all of the time.

I've mentioned the methods by which medical cannabis can be taken according to the current law, and to be more specific, they include:

- Smoking, vaping or intranasal spray
- Orally, with oils, tinctures, and edibles
- Sublingually, with a dropper
- Topicals you apply to the skin, and
- Rectally

Initially, while medical cannabis had been approved in Florida, *smoking* cannabis had not. Prominent Florida attorney John Morgan (of the law firm of Morgan & Morgan) filed a complaint against the State of Florida and a judge in Tallahassee started hearing testimony on whether the legislature acted unconstitutionally in banning the whole plant and the smoking of cannabis. Funny, because as far as smoking a commercially-produced, tobacco-cigarette as opposed to a cannabis-cigarette or "joint," there are carcinogens in one (the Marlboro) and no carcinogens in the other (the joint). Further, the cannabis has CBD in it, which works as an antioxidant and an anti-inflammatory, so it helps protect the lung rather than destroy or demolish the lung, as cigarettes do. The carcinogens, by the way, that appear in commercial cigarettes are from all of the processing that takes place. As a result, there is more than just tobacco in there. There is tar, nicotine, and all kinds of other preservatives and additives. Originally, tobacco was simply grown, dried, then placed in a pipe and smoked. Today there are quite a few additives that are not good for us in them, as we all now know.

There's a valid argument to be made for smoking cannabis. A typical cannabis cigarette or "joint" consists of approximately 0.5 to 1 gram of cannabis and the THC content is approximately 4 percent or 20 mg to 40 mg, respectively. About half of the THC in a joint of herbal cannabis is inhaled in the mainstream smoke. Nearly all of this is absorbed through the lungs, rapidly enters the bloodstream and reaches the brain within minutes. Maximal effect is experienced after 30 minutes and the effect lasts 2-3 hours. This rapid onset and predictable decay allows for effective dosing *not* possible with oral cannabinoids.

Once absorbed, THC and other cannabinoids are rapidly distributed to all other tissues at rates dependent on blood flow. Because they are extremely lipid soluble, cannabinoids accumulate in fatty tissues, reaching peak concentrations in 4-5 days. They are then slowly released back into other body compartments, including the brain. Because of the sequestration in fat, the tissue elimination half-life of THC is about 7 days, and complete elimination of a single dose may take up to 30 days.

In comparing smoked versus vaporized administration, a study found higher serum THC at 30 minutes and 60 minutes post-inhalation with vaporization and comparable serum THC levels over the remaining 6-hour period. Also, vaporization was preferred by 80 percent of the subjects in the study.

The bioavailability after oral ingestion, however, is much less. Blood concentrations reached are 25-30 percent of those obtained by smoking the same dose, partly because of first-pass metabolism in the liver. The onset of effect is delayed (0.5-2 hours) but the duration is prolonged because of continued slow absorption from the gut.

Cannabinoids are highly hydrophobic, making transport across the aqueous layer of the skin the rate-limiting step in the diffusion process. No clinical studies exist regarding the percutaneous absorption of cannabis-containing ointments, creams, or lotions. However, some research has been carried out on transdermal delivery of synthetic and natural cannabinoids using a dermal patch. A patch containing 8 mg of THC suggested an absorption period of 1.4 hours in a guinea pig model, and this concentration was maintained for at least 48 hours.

Cannabis is known to be consumed in baked goods such as cookies or brownies or drunk as teas or infusions. However, absorption of these products by the oral route is slow and erratic, as mentioned previously, and the onset of effects is delayed with the effects lasting much longer compared to vaping. Dosages for orally administered products are even less well established than for vaporization. Dosing remains a highly individualized matter. Patients with no prior experience with cannabis and initiating inhaled cannabis therapy for the first time are cautioned to begin at a very low dose (0.2 mg/kg. for the inexperienced and 0.5 mg/kg. for the more experienced) and to stop therapy if unacceptable or undesirable side-effects occur.

Cannabis has many variables that do not fit well with the typical medical model for drug prescribing; for example:

- The complex pharmacology of cannabinoids
- The inter-individual (genetic) differences in cannabinoid receptor structure and function
- The inter-individual (genetic) differences in cannabinoid metabolism affecting cannabinoid bioavailability
- Pharmacological tolerance to cannabinoids
- Changes to cannabinoid receptor distribution/density and/or function as a consequence of a medical disorder
- The variable potency of the cannabis plant material
- The different dosing regimens and routes of administration used in different research studies all contribute to the difficulty in reporting precise doses or establishing uniform dosing schedules for cannabis and/or cannabinoids

The point? Recommendations for medical cannabis are and should be very individualized and closely monitored matters between you and your medical-cannabis-qualified physician. But becoming a patient is not impossible, in fact with guidance it can be very simple.

According to the Florida Department of Health, Office of Medical Marijuana Use (OMMU), today there are over 200,000 patients in the registry for medical cannabis, over 2,000 qualified physicians who can legally recommend its use, 13 approved medical marijuana treatment centers, and other legal issues are moving forward, such as your ability to grow your own cannabis. Things *are* changing, and as more people find out the truth and find out about the possibilities for cannabis as a natural and effective remedy, the more the lies of the past fall away, and the quicker things change for the better.

In fact, while writing this book, yet another major change has taken place.

[12] CONSUMING CANNABIS

"Of course I know how to roll a joint."
—MARTHA STEWART
TV Personality

EFFECTIVE LATE MARCH 2019, Senate Bill 182 was signed into law by Florida Governor Ron DeSantis. The law states that the medical marijuana treatment centers ("MMTCs" or dispensaries in the United States—in Canada they're called Licensed Producers or "LPs") can now have either pre-rolled marijuana cigarettes (a.k.a. "joints") or they can now supply the dried flower (or "bud"). The flower is being sold in 3.5 to 4-gram packets, which is approximately an eighth of an ounce (one ounce being 28.3495 grams). A

3.5 to 4-gram packet now runs between $33 and $55, depending on the *chemovar* that you're getting. (What has traditionally been called a cannabis *strain*, such as indica, sativa, or hybrid, should really be called a *chemovar* or *subspecies*. People in the industry have often and erroneously used the term *strain*. Strains, however, only occur in bacteria and viruses. Plants on the other hand cannot have a *strain*. In plants you have a *family*, or a *genus*, you have the *species* or the *subspecies*. Nonetheless people have been using the term *strain* to refer to different cannabis *subspecies* or *chemovars*.) The way the law reads now is patients can get a maximum of 2.5 ounces every 35 days.

So we do now in Florida have the *flower* or *bud* available for individuals to smoke or utilize in so many other ways, in addition to the oils we have had up to now. Oils are great, of course, for vaping, for sublingual use, for oral mucosal use in the form of a spray, for inhalation in the form of a nasal spray or an inhaler like the traditional asthma inhalers. Flower can be smoked or it too can be vaporized. You can purchase a hand-held vaporizer *for flower*, and one of the more popular ones is from a company called PAX. Those are cool because you can control the temperature setting of the vaporizer. And that's important because certain cannabinoids have different boiling points and if you use too high of a heat setting you could burn out some of the cannabinoids. But by using a lower heat setting you can utilize and get more of the cannabinoids from the plant. If you visit www.JosephRosadoMD.com you can get a free report that lists and explains all of the most important boiling points for cannabis, as well as boiling points for certain other herbs and plants that can be vaporized for healing purposes. For example, lavender, chamomile, basil, rosemary. All of those can be vaporized together with the cannabis to accentuate the healing properties of the cannabis by utilizing *terpenes* that provide some of the healing properties as well as the smell and the taste, and which aid in the anti-inflammatory properties or assist with relaxation, calming, sleep, energy, and so on.

Another advantage of being able to process the whole flower is that you can utilize it to infuse foods. You can do this either without *decarboxylation* (without "cooking" the bud) or after. I'll explain, because there are advantages to both states of your cannabis. Using raw, dried flower, without heating it first, you get many of the benefits of the cannabis without the euphoria because you're leaving the natural acidic properties of the cannabis intact. The acidic component has a lot of antioxidant properties, has a lot of anti-inflammatory properties, and has anti-cancer properties, with no euphoria. Cannabis flower contains, for example, THCA—which is THC with its natural acid. Ingesting cannabis in this state will provide the added benefits of the acidic component *without* the high or euphoria, which is only accessible after heating the cannabis sufficiently to convert THCA to THC. This is why recreational marijuana has to be heated in order to provide a high, whether that's by smoking or cooking, for example. Heating your cannabis sufficiently to convert THCA to THC is called *decarboxylation*. Before the cannabis is heated to a temperature of 220 degrees Fahrenheit, it has COOH, or *carboxylic acid*. When the plant is heated to 220 degrees or greater for a sufficient amount of time it becomes *decarboxylated*, meaning it loses the acidic property. The CBDA or the THCA or the CBGA, which are the acidic versions of the cannabinoids, will be decarboxylated, leaving CBD, THC, and CBG.

Or, you can use the non-cooked flower and infuse it into oils, like coconut oil or olive oil, and make a dressing for your salad. Or, you can use the flower, the actual bud itself, and chop it up and put that directly into your salad. Or you can use the bud and put it in your juice, if you're a juicer. You can also make teas out of it. By boiling water and then removing the water from the heating element and placing the bud in there and letting it steep for 20 minutes, you can make a phenomenal tea that will aid your relaxation, help you sleep, and so on. You can put some cannabis in a crockpot with whatever oil you like and let it run for about four hours and infuse your oil in this way. Or you can make a pesto sauce. Put in your baby greens and some basil and pine nuts. You can add cannabis to that and put the olive oil in while it's being stirred in your food processor. Because cannabis is lipophilic—it loves fat—it binds to the olive oil.

So, you get a nice edible component with the flower. You can make your own edibles as well—cakes, cookies, brownies, even gummy bears. There are some really great recipes at Leafly.com. (I reference Leafly when I discuss the different subspecies and the different chemovars—the Blue Dream, Pineapple Express, Granddaddy Purple— especially in terms of the percentages of CBD to THC and some of the scientific benefits. In fact last week I was interviewed by Leafly on the subject of cannabis for allergies, as we enter allergy season.)

"I mistakenly believed the Drug Enforcement Agency listed marijuana as a Schedule 1 substance because of sound scientific proof. Surely, they must have quality reasoning as to why marijuana is in the category of the most dangerous drugs that have 'no accepted medicinal use and a high potential for abuse.'

"They didn't have the science to support that claim, and I now know that when it comes to marijuana neither of those things are true. It doesn't have a high potential for abuse, and there are very legitimate medical applications. In fact, sometimes marijuana is the only thing that works …

"We have been terribly and systematically misled for nearly 70 years in the United States, and I apologize for my own role in that."

—Dr. Sanjay Gupta
August 8, 2013, "Why I Changed My Mind on Weed," CNN.com

PART IV:
HEALING

{ 1 } CANCER

"It made me feel like I had an appetite for the first time in probably six months. Instead of lying around thinking about how sick I felt all the time — which was not my personality, which was very upsetting to my whole family — I was up and cooking, which was not anything I had done since I hadn't felt well."

—KATE MURPHY
Cannabis Patient

IT'S NATURAL AND HEALTHY that our cells divide and replace themselves again and again throughout our lives. But when this process goes out of control, and more cells are produced than needed, this is how cancer starts and often results in the presence of a tumor or cluster of such "extra" cells. Not all tumors are cancerous, they can be benign or non-cancerous, but most cancers form tumors. Benign tumors do not spread, rob nutrients from the body, or interfere with healthy body processes as cancerous tumors do. And if a cancer starts spreading to other parts of the body through the lymphatic or blood system, this is called *metastasis*, which is a serious development of the illness, as new tumors can form, and new problems can arise in various parts of the body.

There are currently over 100 known forms of cancer. They can affect all parts of the body and its systems, and they can all be life-threatening. Cancer has plagued man for thousands of years, but it is only in recent years that we have begun to understand the illness and work to prevent and defeat it, however, traditional treatments and their side-effects are famously controversial.

WHAT ARE TRADITIONAL TREATMENTS AND SIDE-EFFECTS?

Most mainstream medical doctors or *oncologists* (those who specialize in cancer) will recommend a treatment plan that includes some or all of the following:

- Surgery. This along with the anesthetics and powerful painkillers needed can have life-threatening consequences and at great financial costs. Nonetheless, there are instances where surgery is the most recommended route or at least an ingredient of one's treatment plan. Surgery is most often recommended if the cancer has not yet spread to other parts of the body.

- Chemotherapy. Using powerful drugs to kill cancer cells is a typical ingredient of a traditional cancer treatment plan. Most chemotherapy is administered through injections, topical creams, or orally. And while side-effects vary, the following are typical:

- o Pain
- o Loss of hair
- o Nausea
- o Vomiting
- o Fatigue
- o Diarrhea
- o Mouth sores
- o And, (in the long-term) nerve damage and infertility

- Radiation. Sometimes radiation is a stand-alone treatment in traditional Western medicine, and sometimes it is part of a larger treatment plan. Often the application of radiation is not painful but can be followed thereafter by fatigue, pain, and rashes on the skin, and other long-term damage to surrounding areas.

- Targeted therapy, wherein drugs are administered to prevent the growth or spread of cancer cells.

- Immunotherapy or biologic therapy, stimulating the body's own immune system so that it overcomes the cancer.

- Hormone therapy against cancers that use hormones to grow such as breast and prostate cancer.

- Stem cell transplants, wherein healthy stem cells are taken from the bone or blood and used to replace those cells killed by other forms of cancer treatment.

- Photodynamic therapy, where drugs are added to the blood and a form of light is used to kill cancer cells.

How Does Medical Cannabis Work for Cancer?

Nausea and Vomiting

Cannabis may be best known for its ability to reduce nausea and vomiting caused by chemotherapy. It's so effective that a pill form of THC (Marinol) has been approved by the FDA for treating chemotherapy-induced nausea and vomiting since 1985.

Weight Loss & Appetite

Along with nausea, patients undergoing chemotherapy often find it hard to maintain normal weight. Cannabis has been shown to not only relieve nausea but stimulate appetite as well. For patients with cancer, cannabis can help improve food intake and prevent unhealthy loss of weight.

Mood

Cancer patients often suffer from mood disorders such as depression. While it's no secret that marijuana makes users feel good, research seems to explain why. As many studies have found, chemicals in cannabis appear to have significant anti-anxiety and antidepressant effects.

Pain

Another well-known effect of cannabis is pain relief. And while its benefits seem to span a range of chronic pain disorders, studies show that cannabis can help reduce pain in cancer as well.

Sleep

Patients with cancer often suffer from sleep problems, including difficulty falling asleep and maintaining sleep. On the other hand, sleepiness is one of cannabis' most commonly reported side-effects. THC has also been shown to improve sleep in patients undergoing chemotherapy.

Fatigue

Cancer-related fatigue can also cause patients to feel sleepy during the day. Interestingly, cannabis seems to help patients combat daytime fatigue, while at the same time helping patients get to sleep at night. It's multi-faceted effect on sleep may depend on the strain of cannabis and the balance of cannabinoids that they contain.

Constipation

Chemicals in cannabis help regulate the digestive system and have been suggested as a treatment for a wide range of bowel disorders. While cannabis seems to help by reducing bowel movements in inflammatory bowel disorders, it appears to have an opposite effect in constipation.

Itching

Itching can be a side effect of various cancers as well as various cancer treatments. While the underlying causes of itching in cancer patients vary, cannabis seems to help some patients deal with this irritating symptom.

General

Perhaps the most promising (and controversial) benefit of cannabis in cancer is the treatment of cancer itself. While preclinical studies have long supported the ability of cannabis to kill cancer cells and stop the disease from spreading, the medical community points out that human research is lacking. Nonetheless, I have seen tumor shrinkage in patients being treated with medical cannabis.

My Experience

I work with all kinds of cancers, from children who have rhabdomyosarcoma, to adults with prostate, breast, lung, astrocytoma/brain, colorectal, pancreatic, the full gamut. I recommend cannabis-based oils, the extract of the plant, for these individuals. I have a few patients that are in remission—they're cancer-free, their tumors have shrunk, their energy levels have gone up, no nausea, no vomiting, no weight loss, none of the side-effects that occur as a result of having chemo and radiation. They do extremely well.

Often the recovery from a regimen of chemo and radiation is as bad or worse than enduring the actual, traditional, "treatment." The people who are easily nauseous, underweight, unhealthy, weak as a result of their traditional, mainstream "treatment" can continue to benefit from medicinal cannabis because it will help replenish their energy. Because of the CBD component it will help reduce and eliminate their inflammation. The antioxidants are going to eat up those free radicals. And the THC is going to help with their state of well-being. It's going to support their appetite and energy, and more.

Treating all of these patients with cannabis is very fulfilling because I have people who, as I said, are in remission. In fact, there are patients I share with a hospital which doesn't participate, doesn't recommend cannabis, doesn't engage in this, of course. The patients return to the hospital after participating in cannabis treatments and then, after testing and examination are told they are doing great, often being told, "See you in a year for your annual PET scan."

Research

There is a wealth of laboratory evidence that suggests cannabis kills cancer cells in a number of ways. We are finding cannabinoids can have the following effects in the treatment of cancers:

- *Antiproliferative* effects, which prevent cancer cells from reproducing.

- *Antiangiogenic* effects. Cancerous tumors need to form new blood vessels in order to grow, which cannabinoids seem to prevent.

- *Antimetastatic* effects, preventing cancer from spreading to other organs.

- *Apoptotic* effects, where cannabinoids speed the death of abnormal cells, while preserving the life of the healthy cells around them.

Something we find very exciting is the fact that cannabinoids have the ability to pass through the blood-brain barrier, making cannabis a promising factor in the battles against brain cancer in particular. And in general, we are finding that when the endocannabinoid system is stimulated by cannabinoids it has an anti-tumor effect. THC injected into brain tumors in mice and rats has shown in labs to reduce the size of the tumors and more research, where allowed, is ongoing.

Case Study

When Kate Murphy (not a patient of mine) was diagnosed with breast cancer at 49 and sought to find out about medical marijuana to alleviate the side-effects of the traditional treatments she was undergoing, she was surprised (and frustrated) by the lack of advice from her mainstream doctors on the subject. But it didn't stop her. She was suffering "non-stop nausea" from her chemotherapy, despite trying everything they were recommending—and cannabis was not among those recommendations. After two months of "therapy" the already-thin Kate lost 15 pounds.

It was while waiting for her first dose of chemo that a fellow patient instructed her to make sure she got some medical marijuana. Kate's home state of Massachusetts had legal medical marijuana for six years at that point, but Kate still found it hard to get basic information about if from her traditional medics, not to mention getting a state-issued medical marijuana card. She was basically left to find things out on her own. Even her oncologist, whom she really likes, had little to offer. A small percent of doctors in Massachusetts (like Florida) are actually trained, knowledgeable, and registered to recommend cannabis. Few take the required instruction, and few decide to confront what backlash and repercussions becoming a "pot doc" can have on one's practice, even if cannabis is a viable remedy for recommendation.

But on her own, Kate did find a knowledgeable and registered doctor for recommending medical cannabis, and a dispensary with medical-grade cannabis products such as cannabis-infused honey, lip balms, and bath bombs. The choices might have overwhelmed Kate, had she not found her cannabis-knowledgeable doctor to make recommendations. Kate tried smoking cannabis and credits an improvement in her state to just a few instances of trying cannabis. "It made me feel like I had an appetite for the first time in probably six months," she said.

She made it through her treatments, and Kate is now cancer-free.

{ 2 } EPILEPSY AND SEIZURES

"I didn't hear her laugh for six months. I didn't hear her voice at all, just her crying. I can't imagine that I would be watching her making these gains that she's making, doing the things that she's doing (without the medical marijuana). I don't take it for granted. Every day is a blessing."

—PAIGE FIGI
Cannabis Patient's Mother

SEIZURES, BY THEMSELVES, are short-term episodes of twitching or jerking, usually in the arms or legs, and not necessarily dangerous, unless of course you happen to be driving or doing something else where a seizure could create a dangerous situation. *Epilepsy,* on the other hand, is a brain disorder that causes unusual electrical activity (in the brain) which in turn causes seizures. Roughly 125,000 Americans are diagnosed with epilepsy every year. Epilepsy and seizures are often regarded as synonymous. You may have someone who has been diagnosed with epilepsy, but then you have someone with Dravet syndrome or Lennox-Gastaut syndrome (LGS) which are seizure disorders but don't fall under the umbrella of epilepsy.

While there is no generally-accepted cause of epilepsy or seizures, there are certain things that can be directly tied to their appearance:

- Infections of the brain
- Alterations to structure of the brain
- Brain tumors
- Blood vessel diseases and strokes
- Head injuries, especially when severe
- And possibly, *genetics,* as seizures and epilepsy sometimes seem to run in families.

Seizures are classified by both where they first appear/where they seem to start in the brain and by their effects. *Focal seizures* begin on one side of the brain. During a "focal aware" seizure, one is awake and able to respond to others during the seizure, as opposed to a "focal impaired" seizure during which one is not completely able to interact or aware of what is going on. "Focal motor seizures" cause the body to twitch, jerk, or make other (involuntary) movements. And "focal non-motor seizures" affect the way one feels or thinks. *Generalized seizures* start on *both sides* of the brain. "Generalized motor seizures" make the body twitch or move, but "generalized non-motor seizures" do not make the body move in any particular way.

One might move involuntarily or have certain unusual feelings when having a seizure, and typically if one has seizures, they tend to be similar in each manifestation, which may include these below. These phenomena can last seconds or for minutes:

- Strange feelings

- Experiencing unusual tastes, sounds, sights, or odors
- Physical tics such as rubbing hands or moving your lips
- Twitching or jerking in the arms or legs
- Passing out
- Disorientation, forgetting where you are
- Staring off into space.

In addition to asking questions about both your mental and physical state before, during, and after seizures your doctor will likely also recommend an EEG[10] to check for unusual electrical activity in your brain, as well as a blood sample to test for infections and other possible causes. He or she may also prescribe a powerful X-ray, called a *CT scan* (computed tomography), taking detailed, interior images of your brain in the hunt for tumors or infection, or an *MRI* (magnetic resonance imaging), making pictures by use of radio waves and magnets, looking for the same. In general, when one has had at least two seizures within any 24-hour period, an epilepsy diagnosis becomes possible.

WHAT ARE TRADITIONAL TREATMENTS AND SIDE-EFFECTS?

As with other major ailments, when discussing epilepsy and seizures, most often the discussion is not about *cures,*

---

[10] An EEG or electroencephalogram is "a test that detects abnormalities in your brain waves, or in the electrical activity of your brain. During the procedure, electrodes consisting of small metal discs with thin wires are pasted onto your scalp. The electrodes detect tiny electrical charges that result from the activity of your brain cells." — www.hopkinsmedicine.org

but about *controlling symptoms*. There are standard, traditional treatments prescribed, including:

- Prescription drugs. This is the main way most doctors work to control seizures in patients. Anti-seizure medications include a long list of brand-name prescriptions, including Valporal, Topamax, Lyrica, Dilantin, Ativan, Neurontin, Depacon, Valium, Klonopin, and Tegretol. Doctors try to match the particular drug with the kind of seizures one is having, but often when one doesn't seem to work, they move on and try another.

- Brain surgery, whereby your doctor removes certain parts of your brain or makes cuts in your brain in an attempt to prohibit seizures.

- Medical devices. There are currently two devices used by doctors to prevent seizures: vagus nerve stimulation (VNS) and responsive neurostimulation (RNS). The first (VNS) sends a regular electrical pulse to your brain, and the device is installed in your chest, just under your skin. The last (RNS) performs much the same way, but the device is inserted under your scalp.

- Diet. The *ketogenic diet* is a low-carb, high-fat regimen that has been found to help control seizures in children and may possibly be of some benefit with adults, too. More research is ongoing.

As far as drawbacks are concerned, with many of these above they would seem obvious. A ketogenic diet can be complicated, unpleasant, and hard to maintain with a child. Devices implanted into the body are costly and of course, undesirable, perhaps even more so with brain surgery. And prescription drugs, of course, are famous for side-effects, which with antiseizure medications can include:

- Tremors
- Blurry vision
- Ataxia (loss of full control of the body—*yes, an antiseizure medication has the side effect of loss of control of the body*)
- Vertigo (sense of whirling or loss of balance)
- Fatigue
- Vomiting
- Headaches
- Nausea
- Dizziness

HOW DOES MEDICAL CANNABIS WORK FOR EPILEPSY AND SEIZURES?

Research

Evidence from laboratory studies, anecdotal reports, and small clinical studies from a number of years ago suggest that *cannabidiol* or CBD, a non- psychoactive compound of cannabis, could potentially be helpful in controlling seizures. In 2012, a literature review of clinical studies on cannabinoids for epilepsy could not give a reliable conclusion about the effectiveness of four randomized controlled trials of cannabidiol (CBD). Yet in the 48 people included in these reports, no side-effects were noted. Conducting studies can be difficult as researchers have limited access to cannabis due to federal regulations and even more limited access to cannabidiol (CBD).

Individual reports of children with refractory (or intractable) epilepsy who have tried cannabis, usually with high ratios of cannabidiol to THC, have reported marked improvements in seizure frequency, including a report describing the results of Charlotte, a girl with Dravet syndrome.

Recently, there have been some open-labeled studies in the United States of Epidiolex (a drug derived from cannabidiol or CBD), which is produced by GW Pharmaceuticals. Epidiolex is a purified, 99 percent oil-based extract of CBD that is produced to give known and consistent amounts in each dose. The U.S. Food and Drug Administration (FDA) has given some epilepsy centers permission to use this drug as "compassionate use" for a limited number of people at each center. Such studies are ongoing for difficult epilepsies such as Lennox-Gastaut syndrome (in children and adults) and Dravet syndrome in children.

Results from 213 people who received Epidiolex (99 percent CBD) in an open label study (without a placebo control) were presented at the American Academy of Neurology, April 22, 2015 in Washington DC. Data from 137 people who completed 12 weeks or more on the drug were used to look at how helpful or effective the drug was. People who received the Epidiolex ranged from 2 to 26 years old with an average age of 11. All had epilepsy that did not respond to currently available treatments—25 in the study or 18 percent had Dravet Syndrome (DS) and 22 or 16 percent had Lennox-Gastaut Syndrome (LGS).

- Seizures decreased by an average of 54 percent in 137 people who completed 12 weeks on Epidiolex.

- Patients who had DS responded more positively, with a 63 percent decrease in seizures over three months.
- This improvement in seizures lasted through 24 weeks on the Epidiolex, more often for people with DS than without DS.
- In 27 patients with atonic[11] seizures (which are commonly seen in people with LGS as well as other types of epilepsy), the atonic seizures decreased by 66.7 percent on average.
- The responder rate (the number of people whose seizures decreased by at least 50 percent) was also slightly better in patients with DS (about 55 percent at three months) as compared to patients without DS (50 percent).
- People who were also taking the anti-seizure medication Clobazam (Onfi) seemed to respond more favorably to the Epidiolex with a greater improvement in convulsive seizures than in patients who were not taking Clobazam. The authors suggested that an interaction between Clobazam and Epidiolex may play a part in the differences seen.
- 14 people withdrew from the study because the drug was not effective for them.

My Experience

I have quite a few children patients who have epilepsy, and many adults as well who have seizures and epilepsy,

---

[11] Atonic seizures are a type of generalized seizure and are more common in children than adults. They involve a sudden loss of muscle tone, making a child go limp and fall to the ground. They are often present in children who also have other seizure types, such as tonic or myoclonic seizures." —www.aboutkidshealth.ca

and I have adults who were on anywhere from three to seven seizure medications, and now are either not on any seizure medication at all or are on maybe one regular seizure medication and one break-through medication for break-through seizures, thanks to cannabis.

Case Study

You may have heard about the now-famous case of little Charlotte Figi, often referred to as "Charlotte's Web," presented by Sandra Young of CNN in 2013 and further popularized by the excellent television special report by Dr. Sanjay Gupta called *Weed.* When Charlotte was just three months old, she had her first seizure. She would soon experience recurring seizures lasting at times for *hours* and was repeatedly being brought to the hospital. "They did a million-dollar work-up," said her mom, Paige, "MRI, EEG, spinal tap . . . and found nothing. And sent us home." All her scans and blood tests were normal, yet the *severe* seizures continued. The Fijis were simply told their daughter would, hopefully, grow out of them.

But the seizures actually got worse, and eventually one doctor suggested this might be Dravet Syndrome, a severe, rare, and intractable (medications having no effect) form of epilepsy. Despite a powerful and addictive regimen of prescription drugs, Charlotte's seizures actually got worse. Finally, after a test in a Colorado hospital, Charlotte was confirmed to suffer from Dravet Syndrome. After starting her on a ketogenic diet, which seemed to help with the seizures, Charlotte started showing serious side-effects including bone loss, immune-system problems, and behavioral problems. And after two years on the special diet the seizures returned.

In November of 2000 Colorado approved Amendment 20, which required the state to create a medical marijuana program for citizens. Prior to their daughter's diagnosis,

Paige had voted *against* medical marijuana, but by now, she and husband Matt were investigating it as an alternative for Charlotte, as she was now having 300 seizures *each week,* and had lost the ability to talk, walk, and even eat. Her heart began to stop at some episodes, and her parents had even signed a DNR (do-not-resuscitate order) with the hospital.

Doctors, meanwhile, believed a high-CBD, low-THC form of cannabis could quiet the electrical and chemical activity which causes seizures, and the Fijis finally decided to give it a try. She was the youngest patient to ever apply for the approval of two doctors to try medical marijuana in the state, and despite their concerns about cannabis use in younger patients (particularly when smoked, although Charlotte would not be smoking it) the risks were clearly small in comparison to those associated with the regimen she had already been through with other medications and diet.

The Figis, terrified, began with a small dose of CBD oil for Charlotte. The seizures stopped. Each hour they waited and expected a seizure, but Charlotte was free of them *for the following seven days.* But the supply of the oil was running out, so the Fijis searched and found the Stanley brothers—sanctioned Colorado growers who had crossbred such a strain of cannabis. They would meet Charlotte, provide her the type of cannabis she needed (now affectionately called "Charlotte's Web"), and begin the Realm of Caring Foundation, providing medical cannabis to people suffering from cancer, epilepsy, MS, and Parkinson's disease, who might otherwise not be able to afford the medicine.

Charlotte began receiving two doses of cannabis oil in her food each day. Her seizures stopped. Said her father, Matt, "I literally see Charlotte's brain making connections that haven't been made in years. My thought now is, why were we the ones that had to go out and find this cure? This natural cure? How come a doctor didn't know about this? How come they didn't make me aware of this?"

{ 3 } GLAUCOMA

"I now vape for nearly instant relief. Before I would have taken pills that would take time to go into effect and still leave me with stomachaches and ulcers . . . I am surprised by what a difference it makes . . . when I add up what I was paying for all my meds (even with copays), Heather (vaporizer oil cartridges; a product with a 1:1 ratio of THC to CBD) winds up being cheaper. It's less harmful to my body and definitely has improved my quality of life."

—ERIN DELANEY
Cannabis Patient

MANY PEOPLE THINK of the "optic nerve" as a *single* nerve connecting the human eye to the brain, along which the input received from the eye is sent along accordingly to the brain. The optic "nerve," however, is a *bundle* of more than one *million* nerve fibers, connecting the light-sensitive tissue at the back of the eye (the *retina*) to the brain. The integrity and health of that "nerve" is vital for good vision.

Glaucoma is a group of diseases that adversely affect that nerve, resulting in loss of vision or even blindness.

Simply, it's *pressure* buildup in the eye that leads to glaucoma. It can be the pressure of fluid buildup in the eye or it can be blood pressure. That said, some of us can handle greater levels of pressure in our blood and in our eyes, and not fall prey to glaucoma, but some of us cannot. So on an individual basis, that level of pressure can vary, but it's when a level of pressure too great to be handled by our eyes is created that we suffer normally from damage to the optic nerve and thus, glaucoma and a partial or entire loss of vision. And some types of people are found to be at greater risk than others, such as:

- Those with a family history of glaucoma
- Anyone over the age of 60, especially Mexican Americans
- African Americans over the age of 40

This said, glaucoma can also develop in the absence of increased pressure of the eye (or blood). This is called "low-tension" or "normal-tension" glaucoma.

WHAT ARE TRADITIONAL TREATMENTS AND SIDE-EFFECTS?

Risk factors for glaucoma can be detected via *comprehensive dilated eye exams,* and if warranted, eye drops can be prescribed which have been found to reduce the risk of acquiring glaucoma by as much as half. This is important (prevention) because glaucoma can develop in one or both eyes initially without symptoms, without pain, and even without any loss of vision. With the onset of glaucoma, however, one might notice the gradual loss of peripheral vision, and eventually, a loss of straight-ahead vision as well, until complete blindness. There is no known cure for glaucoma at this time, and no known way to restore vision once lost.

But the worsening of glaucoma can be slowed, if vision cannot be restored, and there are a few traditionally-accepted methods of treatment:

- Medicine. In the form of eye drops or pills, medicine can be effective if glaucoma is detected and a regimen of treatment begun in its early stages. By either causing the eye(s) to manufacture less fluid or to drain more fluid from the eye(s), the pressure therein can be lowered, preserving and protecting the optic nerve. Such medicines must be taken regularly and are often associated with certain side-effects:

  o Redness
  o Stinging
  o Burning
  o Headaches

  And because glaucoma is often symptom-free, if indicated, drops or pills must be continually taken regularly to prevent the onset or progression of vision loss.

- Trabeculoplasty. With trabeculoplasty an argon laser carefully stretches, by burning, the drainage holes in your eyes. The procedure can cause inflammation, and there is some risk the procedure will *increase* the pressure in the eye. Often medications (drops) still

need to be taken, and the procedure often
needs to be repeated down the road.

- Surgery. If medicines and in-office
  trabeculoplasty fail to help, conventional
  surgery might then be recommended, with
  essentially the same goal, to create larger (by
  cutting) openings through which fluid might
  drain (and thereby release pressure in the eye).
  So you can still see, only one eye can be
  operated on at a time, and surgeries must be
  performed about six weeks apart from each
  other. For weeks after a surgery, medications
  (eyedrops, different than that mentioned
  above) must be applied because of the
  temporary, greater risk of inflammation and
  infection. Conventional surgery is historically
  between 60 and 80 percent effective in the
  reduction of eye pressure. In addition to
  inflammation and infection, risks include
  worsened vision and excessively *lowered* eye
  pressure.

How Does Medical Cannabis Work
for Glaucoma?

The idea that cannabis can be helpful in treating glaucoma
dates to the 1970s. Studies conducted then showed that
smoking cannabis lowered the Intraocular Pressure (IOP)
of people with glaucoma. As a result of this research,
additional studies were conducted examining whether
cannabis or its active ingredient, THC, could be used to
keep IOP lowered. This research was supported by the

National Eye Institute, a division of the National Institutes of Health. The research found that when cannabis is smoked or when a form of its active ingredient is taken as a pill or by injection, it does lower IOP.

My Experience

I have patients with glaucoma. Cannabis has helped with the pressure in their eyes, it's helped with their vision to where they can see better, they use less of the drops they are recommended otherwise, so they are doing better overall.

Case Study

Erin Delaney suffered a traumatic brain injury that left her with a form of glaucoma which is very hard to treat. After exhausting every conceivable other option, Erin decided she was too young to be on "so many pills." It seemed to her specialists that her brain injury was precluding the effectiveness of all prescribed medications, and eventually, after an even more severe attack of pressure—an attack that included pain, nausea, and fear of blindness—led Erin to pursue a new treatment plan.

"If you had told me two years ago," Erin says, "that I would be on medical marijuana, I would have laughed you out of the room. Like many, I thought it was just a bunch of 'pot heads' looking for a legal loophole." But after meeting the highly trained and credentialed staff at her medical marijuana facility she changed her mind. She met the pharmacologist and toured the facilities where the cannabis was grown, oils were extracted, and the medicine prepared. She decided on a vaporized form of cannabis in a 1:1 ratio of THC and CBD, being careful because she also had a seven-year-old to think of.

And within minutes of her first dosing, she felt relief, measuring a seven-point drop in optic nerve pressure, according to her doctor, which also enables further surgery (by keeping her eye pressure low), if she chooses. Using her vaporized form of cannabis has helped Erin reduce the other medications she takes by 50 percent.

{ 4 } HIV AND AIDS

"In addition to the remarkable anti-nausea effects, medical marijuana had one additional benefit–now how do I say this without corrupting the youth of the nation?–I had forgotten how enjoyable it is being stoned. I had forgotten, too, how healing enjoyment can be. Yes, pleasure is therapy. Ease to unravel disease. A deep appreciation of life as an answer to death."

—PETER MCWILLIAMS
Cannabis Patient

HIV, OR *human immunodeficiency virus*, is spread by particular body fluids and attacks the *T cells* of one's immune system. Eventually the virus can attack so many of these cells that the body no longer can defend itself against infections and cancers. Untreated, HIV can lead to AIDS, or *acquired immunodeficiency syndrome*. AIDS is the final stage of HIV and the most severe form of HIV, leaving a patient open to all sorts of *opportunistic* infections. HIV progresses in three particular stages:

1. Acute HIV infection (also called "acute retroviral syndrome" or ARS)
2. Clinical latency
3. AIDS

In the first acute HIV infection stage, within weeks one develops flu-like symptoms, including headaches, body aches and pains, rashes, sore throat, swollen glands, and fevers. During this stage the virus rapidly reproduces in your body, destroying T cells as it does. Gradually, the T cells (or "CD4 cells") may resurge, but not usually to previous levels, leaving one less able to defend against infections and cancers. During this stage, because of the elevated levels of the virus in the blood, you are most at risk for transmitting the disease. It's important to catch the virus at this early stage, if at all possible, and to begin "ART" (*antiretroviral therapy*) as fast as possible.

In the *clinical latency stage* of HIV, the virus is living within the patient without producing symptoms (or producing very mild ones). The average period of this stage for someone *not* on traditional treatment (ART) is actually around ten years but catching the virus and beginning ART at this stage can prolong one's life for decades in cases. But in this stage, one is still liable to spread the disease.

The final and most severe stage of HIV, AIDS, is a state wherein your immune system is so defeated it is unable to defend against most infections. It is generally agreed that when your T cells fall below a certain ratio in your blood, or if you have developed opportunistic infections like oral thrush, Kaposi sarcoma—which are the tumors on the skin, or Pneumocystis jiroveci formerly known as Pneumocystis pneumonia, for examples, you are considered to have AIDS. Survival at this stage is normally limited to three years, or less than one year after a serious infection has been contracted.

WHAT ARE TRADITIONAL TREATMENTS AND SIDE-EFFECTS?

There is currently no known cure for HIV or AIDS, and once acquired, one has it for life. But HIV can be controlled, typically through *antiretroviral therapy* (ART), which was introduced in the mid-1990s, and if begun quickly, a regular regimen can prolong the life of an HIV patient, improve their health, and help prevent the spread of HIV to others. Today in the United States, if ART is employed soon enough, one might live a lifespan that rivals someone without HIV. SO while there is currently no known cure, the disease can be controlled for a long time, if discovered and treated soon enough.

The current and most widely used treatment for HIV, ART, or *antiretroviral therapy,* is based on regular dosage of medications that slow the progression of HIV in the body. These drugs are called *antiretrovirals* (ARV), a variety of which are usually given in combination, and this therapy is called ART. Therapy has reduced the number of AIDS-related deaths over the past decades by reducing the quantity of the virus in the blood, if not eradicating it completely. While modern medications are improving on the number and variety of side-effects, side-effects exist, nonetheless, including:

- Pain
- Fatigue
- Dizziness

- Rashes
- Headaches
- Dry mouth
- Sleep difficulties
- Diarrhea
- Vomiting and nausea

These side-effects can have the bad result of one not taking the medications as regularly as one needs to, and it does occur that the virus may mutate itself in resistance of treatment, making it less effective.

HOW DOES MEDICAL CANNABIS WORK FOR HIV AND AIDS?

While the side-effects of HIV and AIDS treatment can impinge on life quality, studies have shown that medical cannabis can help make the adverse effects more manageable. HIV-positive patients consuming medical cannabis have reported significant improvements in appetite, muscle pain levels, nausea, anxiety, depression, and skin tingling. Studies have found that daily and chronic neuropathic pain related to HIV can be significantly lowered by regular cannabis consumption.

Medical cannabis also boosts appetite and daily functioning, helping to combat weight loss and muscle breakdown. Research also suggests that consuming medical cannabis is safe for patients with HIV/AIDS. One study found no significant association with cannabis use and the CD4 T-cell count of patients co-infected with HIV and HCV, which means medical marijuana had no adverse effects on the immune system.

While research surrounding cannabis' potential treatment effects on the HIV virus itself is ongoing, a recent study discovered that cannabis-like compounds blocked the spread of HIV virus during the infection's late stages. Results from an animal trial also suggest that marijuana might be able to stop the spread of HIV. Monkeys that were infected with an animal form of the virus and administered with THC for 17 months saw a decrease in damage to the immune tissue of the stomach.

My Experience

I have patients with HIV and AIDS. Their wasting syndrome[12] has resolved, they are no longer losing weight, they are gaining weight, their immune systems are building up, their CD4 counts are stable or higher than when they started it, so they are doing much better in that regard.

Case Study

In the last few decades medical cannabis has become very common in the management of HIV and AIDS symptoms, in fact it is said that about *one third* of all HIV and AIDS patients now turn to medical cannabis to mitigate symptoms such as:

- Cachexia (weakness and wasting of the body, "wasting syndrome")

---

[12] "AIDS wasting syndrome isn't a specific disease. Someone with AIDS is said to have it when they've lost at least 10% of their body weight, especially muscle. They may have also had diarrhea for at least a month, or extreme weakness and fever that's not related to an infection." —www.webmd.com

- Loss of appetite
- Pain
- Nausea
- And depression

"Wasting syndrome, in combination with other HIV-related symptoms and conditions," says AIDS patient Daniel J. Kane, "left me thoroughly disabled and desperate to obtain relief. I suffered severe nausea, chronic exhaustion and physical weakness, neurological complications, persistent anxiety, and a total loss of appetite ... I became too ill to ingest the pills that lay at the core of my treatment. Despite my attempts, I simply could not swallow them with any regularity. When I did swallow them, I rarely kept them down."

For about a third of patients who are actively undergoing ART, severe pain is a constant problem. This and other side-effects of ART as said, often discourage patients from prescribed treatment, yet when patients employ medical cannabis into their plan, they are over *three times as likely* to continue treatment, and survival. Keith Vines, an HIV/AIDS patient, states, "I found that it took only two or three puffs from a marijuana cigarette for my appetite to return. Moreover, the beneficial effect took place within minutes rather than hours that I sometimes waited after swallowing a Marinol (a synthetic form of THC) capsule."

And in practice, doctor Neil Flynn has observed, "There is no doubt in my mind that for some seriously ill patients, marijuana can help make the difference between life and death. And that for other terminally ill patients, marijuana can make the difference between exercising control over their final months and days and passing in relative peace and comfort or dying in constant and severe agony."

{ 5 } PTSD
(Post-Traumatic Stress Disorder)

"The cannabis helps mute or lower my negative chatter, which allows for good thoughts and feelings to arise. One veteran, a friend of mine, who recently started using marijuana instead of prescription medication for PTSD, said that with the cannabis, he can feel his emotions, and experience them properly and safely. Before, he just felt numb."

—DIANNA DONNELLY
Cannabis Patient

IN THE PAST, TERMS like "shell shock" or "combat fatigue" were used to describe the often disturbing and intense feelings and thoughts now associated with PTSD, or *posttraumatic stress disorder.* Those disturbing thoughts and feelings can appear long after the traumatic event they witnessed, and come in the form of nightmares and flashbacks, evoking fear, anger, and sadness in the present. Sufferers may avoid triggers or similar people or conditions to the traumatic events (like a soldier who no longer wished to fire a gun), and they may be adversely affected when they are simply touched or hear a loud noise. It's the psychiatric condition that sometimes results from one experiencing the violence of war, an act of terrorism or rape or assault, or even a natural disaster. The condition can arise from a single traumatic event, a chain of them, or even the discovery of such an event when it happens to another.

There are four categories of PTSD symptoms:

1. **Arousal and reactive symptoms**, such as being irritable or having outbursts, easily startled, problems with focus, or reckless or self-destructive.

2. **Negative feeling and thoughts,** particularly about oneself or others, or feelings of detachment, anger, horror, shame, or guilt.

3. **Avoiding triggers,** such as people, places, and certain activities, and avoiding discussing such triggers.

4. **Involuntary and intrusive thoughts,** memories, dreams, flashbacks, and reliving traumatic events.

In the United States today, roughly 3.5 percent of us have been diagnosed with PTSD from various causes, and in our lives, roughly one in eleven of us are destined to be. This odds are twice for women as they are for men. Symptoms can appear right away or months after the trauma witnessed, and can last for weeks, months, or even years. They can be debilitating, interfering with many of life's activities.

WHAT ARE TRADITIONAL TREATMENTS AND SIDE-EFFECTS?

While not everyone who develops PTSD will require professional treatment—some may improve with the help of a support network like friends and family, and some may simply improve over time—many do need professional help in the form of therapy, generally "talk therapy" or medication. Cognitive behavior therapies (CBT) have been found to be effective forms of psychotherapy. There are several types of CBT:

- **Prolonged Exposure Therapy**. In a controlled and safe environment, the patient is run through the details of the traumatic event over and over so as to desensitize the event and learn to cope with what happened.

- **Cognitive Processing Therapy**. A therapist helps the patient confront, understand, and cope with the distressing emotions and memories that currently haunt them.

- **Group and Family Therapy**. It can help to find others that have had similar or the same experience as one that has survived, and to find support in the form of others with such experiences.

In addition to psychotherapy, medication is often resorted to for sufferers of PTSD, at least to control or subdue the symptoms, and sometimes as an aid to psychotherapy. Namely, certain "inhibitors" are often prescribed:

- SSRIs—selective serotonin reuptake inhibitors. Brand names include Lexapro, Prozac, Paxil, and Zoloft. SSRI side-effects can include:
  - o Blurry vision
  - o Headaches
  - o Sexual problems
  - o Dizziness
  - o Agitation
  - o Nervousness
  - o Diarrhea
  - o Insomnia
  - o Dry mouth
  - o Nausea
  - o Drowsiness
  - o And anyone taking anti-depressants will be warned of the associated risk of suicide as well.

- SNRIs—selective norepinephrine reuptake inhibitors. SNRI side-effects can include:
  - o Sexual problems
  - o Appetite loss
  - o Headaches
  - o Problems urinating
  - o Constipation
  - o Agitation
  - o Anxiety
  - o Insomnia
  - o Fatigue
  - o Sweating
  - o Dry mouth
  - o Nausea
  - o Dizziness

- As well as other medications to control anxiety, depression, nightmares, physical agitation, and sleep disorders.

We are about to discuss the use and effectiveness of medical cannabis, of course, but alternative therapies are being used more and more, especially in light of the side-effects listed above, such as acupuncture and animal therapy.

HOW DOES MEDICAL CANNABIS WORK FOR PTSD?

Dr. Raphael Mechoulam has discussed his experiments demonstrating the neuroprotective effects of the endocannabinoid system in mice that have had traumatic injuries to the brain. Another fascinating discovery, one with implications for PTSD, is that the cannabinoid system is integrally related to memory, specifically to memory extinction. Memory extinction is the normal, healthy process of removing associations from stimuli. Dr. Mechoulam explained that an animal which has been administered an electric shock after a certain noise will eventually forget about the shock after the noise appears alone for a few days. Mice without cannabinoid systems simply never forget— they continue to cringe at the noise indefinitely. This has implications for patients with PTSD, who respond to stimuli that remind them of their initial trauma even when it is no longer appropriate. By aiding in memory extinction, cannabis could help patients reduce their association between stimuli (perhaps loud noises or stress) and the traumatic situations in their past.

My Experience

I have *many* patients with PTSD—lots of veterans, both male and female, who have gone through combat or have been raped or mugged or had near-death experiences that have triggers that set them off with post-traumatic stress disorder. With cannabis, they are now doing great. Wives come in and tell me how they've gotten their husbands back. Others come in and tell me how before cannabis they could not leave the house, could not go to a grocery store, and now they go to Disney World. Many people don't understand what a big deal that is for people with PTSD. You're walking into an amusement park that has *thousands of people* pushing, shoving, children crying, and they are now able to go into that kind of environment and they are fine. That means they are now able to be a dad or a mom, they are able to go and do things they were unable to do before.

Case Study

Marijuana for Trauma is a Canadian medical marijuana company specifically for helping military veterans in Edmonton, Alberta, owned and operated by Fabian Henry, who uses it himself to treat his trauma from a tour of duty in Afghanistan. He states that in his experience the conventional medications simply suppress feelings and emotions, but medical cannabis allows one to *process* such trauma. Others claim it helps quiet the noise and self-chatter associated with PTSD, while not going "numb" from prescription drugs. Veteran Program Coordinator for Canadian Cannabis Clinics explains, "Medical cannabis is used in conjunction with other therapies . . . Medical cannabis strains with the right CBD and THC levels are assisting veterans with chronic physical pain, as well as anxiety and insomnia issues. I believe that medical cannabis will continue to work in conjunction with many other therapies."

{ 6 } ALS

(Amyotrophic Lateral Sclerosis)

"Cathy Jordan has consulted with more than 30 neurologists, and none have told her to stop smoking marijuana, which has successfully treated her condition for about two decades, her husband said."

—*TAMPA BAY TIMES*

ALS, OR *AMYOTROPHIC lateral sclerosis,* is a disease that attacks nerve cells in the brain and spinal cord. It was discovered by neurologist Jean-Martin Charcot in 1869. The term means literally, "no muscle nourishment," and ALS results in progressive deterioration of the muscles as it kills motor neurons. As the muscles waste away, certain areas of the spinal cord degenerate, leading to a hardening (or sclerosis) of those areas. Progressively, with greater nerve damage, the patient is less and less able to control and move their muscles. Ultimately this leads to an inability to eat, speak, and even breathe.

There are two types of ALS—*sporadic* and *familial.* Ninety to ninety-five percent of all cases in the United States are *sporadic,* which can affect anyone. The *familial* form is apparently passed down from parents. ALS currently affects more than 20,000 people in the United States, usually between the ages of 40 and 70. It is perhaps most well-known and visible for affecting famous New York Yankee Lou Gehrig and physicist Stephen Hawking, and others.

WHAT ARE TRADITIONAL TREATMENTS AND SIDE-EFFECTS?

ALS can be difficult to diagnose because it resembles other neurological diseases. But tests used to determine the possibility of ALS include electromyograms (EMG, a test of electrical activity using needles inserted into the muscles), nerve conduction studies (to determine if nerve damage exists), magnetic resonance imaging (MRI, using radio waves and a magnetic field to create images of the brain and spinal cord), blood and urine tests (in part to rule out other diagnoses), spinal taps (removing spinal fluid with a small needle for testing), and a muscle biopsy (removing a small amount of muscle for laboratory testing in particular to rule out other ailments). There is currently no known cure for ALS. Efforts then are made to ease the suffering of an ALS patient, either through physical assistance or group and individual support.

Currently treatment does not exist that can stop ALS, but symptoms can be slowed, and the patient can be made as comfortable and independent as possible. There are two medications approved by the FDA:

- **Riluzole**. A pill that slows the progression of ALS in some patients, likely by reducing the

levels of the chemical messenger glutamate.
Side-effects include:
- o Liver problems
- o Gastrointestinal problems
- o Dizziness

- **Edaravone**. An intravenously delivered drug that has shown some promise in slowing the progression of ALS. Side-effects include:
  - o Bruising
  - o Hives
  - o Shortness of breath
  - o Swelling
  - o Problems with gait

Other issues one may have as a result of having ALS include:

- Cramps and spasms
- Outbursts of laughter or crying
- Problems sleeping
- Depression
- Pain
- Phlegm
- Salivation
- Fatigue
- Constipation

As a result, treatment can include therapy for breathing, physical therapy, occupational therapy (to help one remain as independent as possible), speech therapy, nutrition, and psychotherapy.

How Does Medical Cannabis Work
for ALS?

An article titled, "Cannabis Use in Palliative Care," published in the *Journal of Clinical Nursing*, recounts studies that have explored cannabis as a therapy for ALS patients. Carter and Rosen (2001) and Amtmann et al. (2004) suggested that it may be of use in ALS based on studies of other patient groups, particularly those with MS (multiple sclerosis), for whom cannabis acted as an analgesic, muscle relaxant, bronchodilator, saliva reducer, appetite stimulant, sleep inducer and antidepressant. Carter and Rosen also made the point that emerging evidence suggests cannabis has strong antioxidant and neuroprotective benefits, which may prolong cell survival- a key issue for ALS and MS patients, who suffer from the death of motor neuron cells. An online survey conducted by Amtmann found cannabis to be moderately effective in reducing appetite loss, depression, pain, muscular spasticity, drooling and weakness for ALS patients, with the longest relief reported for depression.

My Experience

I do have one patient with ALS. I am waiting on her to get back to me with a report, however, I know of one patient who has had ALS for 35 years, and she is the longest living ALS sufferer in the country, and she attributes her success to the fact that she has been using cannabis all this time.

Case Study

Cathy Jordan of Parrish, Florida, was diagnosed over 30 years ago with ALS. She and her husband spent over five years fighting for medical cannabis in Florida, and since granted in 2016, they have been fighting for cannabis to be permitted in smoking form, the only way she can successfully assimilate the remedy. The constitutionality of the ban on the smoked form is, at this writing, being argued in the courts. In Cathy's case, her home had even been raided by deputies who confiscated cannabis plants, but charges were never brought after Cathy's lawyer successfully showed she needed the plants for treatment of her disease. Cathy must smoke cannabis because she is unable to take it in vapor form, which can make her gag, and if she gags it can kill her, potentially.

Meanwhile, the Jordans attribute Cathy's very survival to her use of medicinal cannabis.

{ 7 } CROHN'S DISEASE

"I've talked to people around the world about cannabis and have been to countless camps for kids with Crohn's disease who don't even know what the word 'remission' is. It feels amazing to explain what cannabis is, how it can help and change their lives."

—COLTYN (17)
Cannabis Patient

CROHN'S DISEASE IS AN inflammation of your digestive system, usually of the colon small intestine, but it can affect any part of the digestive system. Along with *ulcerative colitis,* it is one of several diseases classified as *inflammatory bowel disease.* Symptoms can appear and be severe or not appear at all for weeks or months *or even years* at a time. Depending on where the Crohn's is located and upon the severity, symptoms might include:

- Often bloody, chronic diarrhea, at times with mucus or pus
- Weight loss
- Fever
- Abdominal pain
- Bloated abdomen
- Bleeding from the rectum

The adverse effects of Crohn's can be either local, affecting just the intestines, or *systemic,* affecting the entire body. *Local* complications can include:

- Pockets of pus called **abscesses** in the walls of the intestine
- If your body cannot absorb fat adequately, **bile salt diarrhea**
- Painful tears in the lining of the anus called **fissures**
- Openings that connect two parts of your intestines called **fistulas**
- An inability to absorb nutrients leading to **malabsorption** and **malnutrition**
- Bacteria growth higher up in the digestive tract than normal (small intestine bacterial overgrowth or SIBO), causing bloating, pain, gas, and diarrhea.
- Inflammation that leads to thickening of parts of your intestine called **strictures,** causing blockages, cramps, bloating, and pain.

Systemic complications can include:

- Arthritis
- Skin problems
- Bone loss

- Vitamin D deficiency
- Eye problems
- Kidney problems
- Liver problems
- Growth problems

WHAT ARE TRADITIONAL TREATMENTS AND SIDE-EFFECTS?

There is currently no known cause and no known cure for Crohn's disease. It is known that Crohn's is a chronic inflammation, and not a problem with the immune system, as previously thought. There are factors that can make you more prone to Crohn's, such as genetics, age, and diet. Overuse of medications like ibuprofen and smoking may not cause Crohn's but can certainly make it worse. As with other incurable diseases, treatments focus, then, on alleviating symptoms.

Medications

In the case of Crohn's this means primarily treatment with medications:

- **Anti-inflammatory drugs**, with which side-effects include headaches, nausea, diarrhea, rashes, and upset stomach
- **Corticosteroids,** which are more powerful anti-inflammatory drugs and if taken for more than three months they can cause a wide range of side effects

- **Immune system modifiers,** which can take months to work and create higher risk of life-threatening infections
- **Antibiotics,** side-effects include numbness in the hands and feet, nausea, tears in the Achilles tendon, and a metallic taste in the mouth
- **Diarrhea drugs**
- Other medicines and their accompanying side-effects.

Often a battery of drugs are prescribed and once remission is achieved a maintenance regimen is put in place.

Surgery

When medications do not help as hoped, which is the case in about 75 percent of all cases, surgery is done to address symptoms. Your surgeon may remove the diseased part of the bowel and then reattach the two ends again. This is called **anastomosis,** and while it can create a symptom-free patient for years, it is still not a permanent cure. In fact, Crohn's often returns to the very area of the surgery. If your rectum is diseased your surgeon may attach your intestine to the skin of your torso and attach a bag or pouch that will collect waste. This is called an **ileostomy.**

HOW DOES MEDICAL CANNABIS WORK FOR CROHN'S DISEASE?

While much clinical research is still needed to validate and confirm the great anecdotal evidence thus far, a particular study done in Israel shows great promise for cannabis as used to alleviate Crohn's and its positive results in mitigating inflammation. In a small (but now rather famous) study, 21 Crohn's patients who did not respond to other therapies were studied. Half were given cannabis cigarettes twice a day, while the other half given placebo cigarettes with nonactive ingredients. After ten weeks of the study:

- Of the 11 patients given cannabis, 5 achieved complete remission from Crohn's
- Of the 10 patients given placebos, 1 achieved complete remission from Crohn's.

The study clearly suggest more research is warranted.

My Experience

I have a group of patients who have Crohn's, who have been receiving infusions for many years, and they now no longer have to receive the intravenous infusions. Their discomfort is now under control. As a result, they are not experiencing the same amount of pain as they did before. Their bowel movements are under control. They can leave the house and not be fearful or concerned where previously their outings were dictated by which bathrooms were nearby. By engaging and using cannabis, they now no longer need to be in that situation.

Case Study

Through a few degrees of separation, a colleague of mine was familiar with a family which included a teenager with severe Crohn's disease. After years of frustration and side-effects with conventional medications, they turned to medical cannabis, mostly in vaporized form. The results were dramatic and obvious enough for the family, that the mother became quite adept at gathering—illegally, of course—not only the "flower" of the cannabis plant but the leaves and stems as well. She became skilled at cultivation and preparations for her son, including owning an expensive vaporizing machine, and making cookies, butter, and other edibles for her son to use. She became an advocate, in fact. After they left Florida (but prior to legalization of cannabis for medical use), she apparently also became a sort of Robin Hood—a phenomenon not uncommon in the homes of those who suffer but are prohibited still from legal access to medicinal cannabis— providing low-THC, high-CBD forms of cannabis to families without legal access or funds enough for treatment of their children's seizures, a family member's cancer, and so on.

So it was with great interest I found the following anecdotal study of 14-year old Coltyn, a sufferer of severe Crohn's, whose family moved to Colorado (an early adopter of medicinal cannabis) in the interest of their son's health and well-being. In an article posted exactly a year ago titled, "I'm 17, and Medical Marijuana Is Keeping Me Alive," they explain how Coltyn and his dad left the rest of the family in Illinois to travel to Colorado in search of hope and healing. They had no exact plan, they just felt they had to go, to seek out some kind of answer to Coltyn's Crohn's, feeling they had exhausted all other options. A near-death drowning led to a serious infection that a year later seemed to lead to a diagnosis of Crohn's. After conventional "intense medications and treatments" Coltyn seemed to only get worse and draw back from life and suffer weakness and intense pain. The next wave of "treatments," including drug infusions, led to arthritis, lupus, and serum sickness (wherein a body defends against medications). A switch in medications then led to nosebleeds and a swollen face, fatigue, joint pain, and deterioration of Coltyn's bones. Then according to the family, the prescribed Humira led to a scare that he had contracted tuberculosis or T-cell lymphoma. Coltyn was left weak, underweight, unable to stand or walk, and in a wheelchair. Doctors recommended other powerful drugs, surgery that would leave him permanently with a colostomy bag, or alternative medicine.

They—perhaps *finally*—considered cannabis. "I didn't have much to lose," says Coltyn. A study they found from Israel suggested cannabis might help with Crohn's disease. Coltyn recalls, ". . . when my parents told me that from what they knew, cannabis oil doesn't have any known side-effects, I was on board. Before we looked into cannabis, I was just told it was bad and that I should stay away from it. But I had faith in my parents. They had seen me go through so much." After searching for the best doctors recommending cannabis in Colorado at the time, they decided upon two (as required in Colorado at the time), and Coltyn became the first registered pediatric medical marijuana user for Crohn's in Colorado.

They tried cannabis in brownies. Coltyn remembers, "After the first few weeks, I started feeling better. But I will never touch a brownie again, whether it's medicated or not. I had to eat about two every day for a month." And after a good deal of trial and error, the family had arrived at a workable dosage and a ratio of 1:1 of THC and CBD, and that capsule form worked best to deliver the cannabis to the gut. "After the first three years of pharmaceutical medication, all the doctors were trying to do was mask my disease. I really wanted to find a solution that would help me, and cannabis not only relieved the pain, but it also relieved the inflammation in my intestines and stopped my Crohn's from having flares," he says. "Now nutrients I eat are absorbed, so I have energy and can grow."

And after seven months of medicinal cannabis, Coltyn had a colonoscopy that showed no Crohn's disease, no ulcers, no inflammation, along with healthy blood work. Today, Coltyn has gained weight to a healthy level and is an active young man.

{ 8 } PARKINSON'S DISEASE

1:37 p.m.

Doctor: "The best way to take it, is to put it under your tongue and rub it in your cheek."

Patient: (Sitting on couch, shaking badly, struggles and self-administers cannabis oil.)

Doctor: "Don't do too much or you'll be asleep all afternoon. You know what you should do? Don't try to communicate, just relax, see what happens."

1:39 p.m.

Patient: (Lying on couch, arm behind head, relaxed.)

1:41 p.m.

Patient: (Sits up, no longer shaking.)

Doctor: "I think you've calmed down."

Patient: "So quickly."

Doctor: "Isn't it amazing?"

Patient: (Holds out hands, no longer shaking but stable.) "My voice is coming back."

Doctor: "Okay, it works most of the time."

Patient: (Pauses, thinks, then sings.) "In fact, it's, *Aaaaah!* (laughter) Did you guys eat lunch?"

Doctor: "Are you hungry now?"

Patient: (Sitting stably, smiling.) "Funny, I am. A person like me could really use marijuana. It makes me pretty angry that I can't get it in my home state." (Stands up, stable, holding cane but not using it.)

—YouTube

"Man with severe Parkinson's disease tries Marijuana for the first time"

PARKINSON'S DISEASE was discovered (and named after) English doctor James Parkinson, who first described it in 1817, in "An Essay on Shaking Palsy." A red tulip is the adopted symbol for the disease. In modern times, the disease has been made well-known by public figures who have contracted it, including boxer Muhammad Ali, actor Michael J. Fox, and most recently, actor Alan Alda.

Parkinson's disease (PD) is a disorder that affects certain parts of the brain and progressively gets worse, gradually resulting in body tremors, *bradykinesia* (slowness of movement, one of the primary manifestations of Parkinson's Disease), stiffness of limbs, shaking, and stance and balance problems. These symptoms generally get worse slowly, over a matter of years. Despite these dramatic changes in a person, Parkinson's is not fatal. The complications that arise from having Parkinson's can be life-threatening, however, and complications form PD is the 14th leading cause of death in the United States, at the time of this writing. Specifically, Parkinson's disease is a *neurodegenerative disorder* that attacks dopamine-producing neurons in a particular area of the brain. There are few neurons that produce dopamine as it is, so as the disorder attacks these neurons it can have serious consequences for the patient. Dopamine is a *neurotransmitter,* so the loss of this precious material produces devastating effects as the brain loses its ability to receive information and send commands throughout the body, resulting in cases as the symptoms described within Parkinson's disease.

PD is well-known for the *motor problems* it causes, as described briefly above, but even more significant, perhaps, are the *non-motor* symptoms, which include depression, constipation, sleep problems, cognitive impairment, and loss of the sense of smell. In the advanced stages, dementia is often also a problem. PD usually affects people over the age of 60 and affects men more often than women, with a life expectancy after diagnosis of between 7 and 14 years.

WHAT ARE TRADITIONAL TREATMENTS AND SIDE-EFFECTS?

There is currently no known cure and no known cause (although genetics and environmental factors are suspected), but medication and surgery are often attempted. As PD affects the patient's dopamine levels, there are drugs ("dopaminergic medications") that attempt to replace or alleviate the symptoms of this loss. Regardless, while medications and surgery are often attempted, traditional medicine admits to having no ability to cure PD or even slow its progression, and the focus is often, then, as to how to alleviate symptoms, as with other currently incurable diseases. Interestingly, in the case of PD, there does seem to be some correlation between getting PD if you have a family member with it, if you've been around many pesticides, or if you've had a head injury. And conversely, some research suggests you may be less likely to get PD if you are a tobacco smoker or coffee or tea drinker.

Part of the major problem with PD today is that significant neuron/dopamine loss has usually occurred by the time symptoms become manifest. Therefore, a current focus in research is earlier detection of PD. Meanwhile, common medications include the *antiparkinson medication levodopa* (L-DOPA), although as the disease progresses medications become less effective. When drugs are ineffective surgery is often resorted to. Diet and types of therapy seem to have some positive effect upon symptoms.

Side-effects of levodopa and other Parkinson's medications include:

- Nausea
- Vomiting
- Irregular heart rhythm
- Increased odds for involuntary movements
- Restlessness
- Confusion
- Falling down

HOW DOES MEDICAL CANNABIS WORK FOR PARKINSON'S DISEASE?

Researchers have shown enthusiasm to study cannabis in relation to Parkinson's after people with PD gave anecdotal reports and posted on social media as to how cannabis reduced their tremors. Some researchers think that cannabis might be neuroprotective—saving neurons from damage caused by Parkinson's. Besides reducing tremor, cannabinoids have also been studied for use in treating other symptoms, like bradykinesia (slowness caused by PD) and dyskinesia (excess movement caused by levodopa-one of the medications used to treat PD). People with PD have less CB1 receptors than people who do not have PD. A boost to the CB1 receptor through a substance like cannabis can improve tremors and may alleviate dyskinesia. Similarly, the other receptor, CB2, is also being studied to determine if it can modify the disease or provide neuroprotective benefits, as with ALS and MS.

My Experience

We know from experiments boosting certain branches of the endocannabinoid system is helpful in relieving symptoms of Parkinson's disease. And we know from anecdotal information that certain patients who smoke marijuana experience relief of their symptoms. I have a handful of patients with Parkinson's and their tremors are now under control. They are now able to drive, to play golf, they are able to enjoy life!

Case Study

The dialogue and description from the video that opens this chapter was taken from a YouTube video of a former police officer named Larry Smith, who has, by now, been featured in a series of videos discussing the relief he has found from medical cannabis for his Parkinson's disease. After fighting Parkinson's for over 20 years and trying (enduring) every traditional treatment—*including brain surgery*—Larry finally found a combination of exercise and medical cannabis. And now, to raise awareness, to share his own story of hope and healing, Larry is making a film about his 300-mile bike ride across the state of South Dakota:

https://www.facebook.com/ridewithlarry/

Larry Smith served as a law enforcement officer for 26 years before retiring in 1999, and he tells the story of his 20-year battle with PD in the (upcoming) documentary, *Ride with Larry* (currently lobbying Netflix).

People like Larry are inspirational. They prove not only the efficacy of medical cannabis, but the power and joy of the human spirit, when it decides and seeks out hope and healing in all its various forms.

{ 9 } MS AND CHRONIC MUSCLE SPASMS

"I had severe excruciating pain from muscle spasms, but the muscles themselves aren't to blame. It's coming from damage on my spine and the muscle relaxers and pain pills go right to the muscle itself. Cannabis reduces inflammation, slowing down the disease activity and calming your entire system. It truly saved my life when my doctor ran out of answers. My miracle plant."

—CAROLYN KAUFMAN
Cannabis Patient

THE HUMAN CENTRAL NERVOUS system (CNS) is comprised of the brain and spinal cord. Nerve fibers (called *axons*) are normally protected by *myelin,* a fatty layer of insulation that allows nerve signals to be conducted properly. With multiple sclerosis, immune cells become overactive and damage the myelin sheathing, which results in loss of myelin along with damage to the nerve fibers. Where there is damage there eventually forms lesions or plaque and hardened scar tissue called *sclerosis*. And where the sclerosis occurs there is a loss of the nerve's ability to communicate throughout the body. Signals from the brain along the spinal cord to various parts of the body get stopped or distorted.

While no two people will have the same exact condition with MS, there are common symptoms that patients often have to live with, including:

- Fatigue
- Problems walking
- Tingling or numbness
- Involuntary muscle spasms, especially in the legs
- Stiffness
- Weakness
- Problems with vision
- Dizziness
- Bladder problems
- Sexual problems
- Constipation
- Pain
- Depression and mood swings
- Speech problems
- Problems swallowing
- Uncontrollable shaking
- Seizures
- Problems breathing
- Itchiness
- Headaches
- Loss of hearing

WHAT ARE TRADITIONAL TREATMENTS
AND SIDE-EFFECTS?

There is no known cause for MS, although doctors tend to believe there are a combination of factors that lead to it, including immune system causes, viral and other infections, environmental causes, and genetic causes. While anyone can apparently get MS, it is more common in women than men by a ratio of 3:1, and it is more common in Caucasians than in Hispanics and African Americans, and it is in fact pretty rare in Asians. The most common age range when people seem to receive the diagnosis when they do lies between 20 and 40 years of age. The risk does seem to be higher for those who have family members who also have MS. And in the United States there are over one million people living with MS today.

Treatment, then, focuses mainly on recovery from attacks, slowing the progression of the disease, and managing symptoms. (In the very mildest forms of MS treatment might not be undertaken at all.) For treating attacks of MS, oral medications or intravenous infusions of *corticosteroids* may be employed, to reduce inflammation of the nerves. Side-effects include:

- Insomnia
- Raised blood pressure
- Mood swings

Or one may have one's plasma removed from one's blood and replaced by a protein solution. This method is normally undertaken when steroids have been ineffective.

Otherwise, depending on the type and severity, there exists a long list of medications used to manage symptoms and progression of MS, but there are usually as long a list of side-effects:

- Flu-like symptoms
- Low blood pressure
- Fever
- Nausea
- Increased risk of cancer
- Diarrhea
- Headaches
- Blurred vision

Other than medications, people do undergo physical therapy or take muscle relaxants, and of course, there is hope with medical cannabis for relief today as well. For MS patients, cannabis can have significant anti-inflammatory, antioxidative, antiemetic, antipsychotic, and neuroprotective effects. Further, the CBD component seems to help MS patients reduce pain, fatigue, and spasticity, and improve their mobility. In fact about 77 percent of those studied stated they felt cannabis was helpful in their management of MS symptoms, and the reported no side-effects from its use. Seventy percent stated their quality of life had improved with medical cannabis and stated as well that they were able to reduce their use of other medications.

HOW DOES MEDICAL CANNABIS WORK FOR MS AND CHRONIC MUSCLE SPASMS?

Research is starting to bear out that cannabis can have positive results with a patient's pain and spasticity when they have MS.

My Experience

"Chronic muscle spasms" was one of the original diagnoses specified as okay for cannabis by Florida law. I have patients who have muscle spasms because of multiple back injuries, auto accidents, or chronic muscle spasms due to multiple sclerosis, for example, where they've gotten extremely phenomenal results to where they are able to walk. Same thing with cerebral palsy, that's another condition that causes severe muscle spasms, where they are finally able to walk and move around due to medicinal cannabis. Under this umbrella we might include cerebral palsy, multiple sclerosis. Chronic, non-malignant pain due to back injuries, herniated discs, back surgery, these can all fall under this heading of chronic muscle spasms as well. Also, movement disorders like Huntington's Disease, these would fall under the muscle spasms arena as well.

Case Study

Carolyn Kaufman is an MS advocate who was first diagnosed with MS in 2009, and she believes cannabis has made all the difference for her. Like others cited in this book, she too exhausted all other traditional avenues before finally arriving at medical cannabis and other all-natural approaches to improve her condition. She details her journey—and her loss of 150 pounds—on her weblog, www.withouttheweight.com. But when it comes to her incorporating medical cannabis into her program, states, "When the pain was severe, cannabis was my gift from the earth. It worked when nothing else would. After never smoking before, I used cannabis to come off of all of my symptom management medications."

"Marijuana clearly has medicinal value. Thousands of seriously ill Americans have been able to determine that for themselves, albeit illegally. Like my own family, these individuals did not wish to break the law, but they had no other choice. The numerous attempts to legitimately resolve the issue-via state legislation and federal administrative hearings-have too often been ignored or thwarted by misguided federal agencies. Several states conducted extensive, and expensive, research programs which demonstrated marijuana's medical utility-particularly in the treatment of chemotherapy side-effects. Francis L. Young, the chief administrative law judge of the United States Drug Enforcement Administration, ruled marijuana has legitimate medical applications and should be available to doctors."

—LYN NOFZIGER
Former Press Secretary to Ronald Reagan
Foreword in 1999 book, *Marijuana RX: The Patients' Fight for Medicinal Pot*, by Robert C. Randall and Alice M. O'Leary

CONCLUSION: HOPE

"Herb is the healing of a nation, alcohol is the destruction."

—BOB MARLEY
Legendary Reggae Musician

YOUR FAMILY MEDIC isn't necessarily prepared for everything, as you might think they are. They may very well be untrained or even unaware of the benefits of natural alternatives for alleviation and curing of disease. It's not only the medical schools, it's also the regulating bodies that have been infiltrated or wholly taken over by vested interests, often against anything holistic or natural. But things are changing. The grassroots groundswell for legal cannabis still grows. Do we regulate broccoli? No, we don't. There is no regulation on the amount of broccoli you can grow, or buy, or eat. And like broccoli, cannabis is a *plant*. Of course, there is the psychoactive component to cannabis, but so is there as well with coffee or cocoa plants, given the presence of substances that alter our physiology (and in general, a similar lack of serious side-effects).

And let's not forget you've got something that's completely legal in all 50 states, that doesn't have any psychoactive component and comes from the cannabis plant, which is CBD, cannabidiol. In June of 2014, Senate Bill 1030 was signed into law by the governor. In there, all they made available was the low-THC form of cannabis, and only for four diagnoses:

- Epilepsy
- Chronic conditions that cause seizures
- Chronic conditions that cause muscle spasms
- Cancer

That was the original. law. Two years later they added the Right to Try Act, which allowed the use of medical cannabis which included CBD *and THC* to treat individuals with terminal cancer. However, at the time that both laws were signed, June of 2014 and June of 2016, there was *still no product available* in the State of Florida for me to recommend to anyone. It wasn't until August of 2016 that the first batches were made available by two dispensaries. Three months later we had availability to medical cannabis. And those were my two firsts. In August I was the first to recommend high-CBD, low-THC to a female with brain cancer, and three months later I was the first in the state to recommend full medical cannabis to a pediatric patient.

The restrictions are falling away, wholesale, state-by-state, at least little-by-little. At this writing there are 33 medical-legal cannabis states. Today cannabis is still registered *federally* as a "Schedule 1" narcotic, equal to heroin. But remember, the current opiate epidemic started with physicians writing prescriptions for opiates! And as pharmacies and doctors stop prescribing them, patients go to the streets and buy a $10 bag to satisfy their opiate addiction by buying heroin. Yet the virtually-side-effect-free and all-natural form of cannabis is still opposed at a federal level, if not among many of the states today. I equate this with gay marriage. Until there is someone in the White House who says, "I'm going to make this legal," it will continue to be the way it is. That will likely be the coalescence of legislation at the state and federal level, and bring legalization beyond its tipping point in the U.S. I would liken our current cannabis situation to the prohibition era in the early 20th century. I suspect people in 50 or 100 years will view our time prohibiting cannabis use this same way, as *overreach.*

When legal, regulated, and taxed appropriately, there is incredible potential. States that have embraced legal medical cannabis already are demonstrating absolutely phenomenal results, both in health and in revenue for the state. But the immediate future is still challenging. At this writing, there are barely 2,000 doctors who are certified to do this in the state of Florida. That number may from time to time go down because many doctors, despite their initial interest, once they see the challenges involved, choose not to continue. It's helped my practice, ironically, but it's evidence of the difficulties that still exist in advocating for cannabis, despite the lack of side-effects and the good results, which of course is why I'm so passionate and have decided to be something of a pioneer in this field.

Down the road, the talk is about going recreational, eliminating the whole medical component, which complicates things. From what I hear, the states where they have both medical and recreational cannabis legalized, the medical dispensaries are pretty full, and people still gravitate towards the medical, particularly those that have zero experience with the use of cannabis. And because they have zero experience they need a lot more hand holding and a lot more expertise in helping them with what is going on. I am of the belief that in the year 2020, with the Regulate Florida (www.regulateflorida.com) group in Florida pushing aggressively, and with attorney John Morgan supporting financially, the passing of adult recreational use in the State of Florida will more than likely pass.

The stigma that exists in many people's minds when it comes to recreational cannabis—the tie-dyes and outdoor music festivals, the propaganda, the couch potatoes—unfortunately stands in the way, to some degree, of not only the legitimate research and use of cannabis as medicine, but even of people being open to it as a treatment in the first place. Busting that stigma, or at least separating medical use and research out from recreational use, which is a whole other matter, is part of my purpose in preparing this book. Volusia County, for example, is a real stickler about government employees using medical cannabis. They still have zero tolerance for it. That said, I have had some schoolteachers tell me their school board has now told them that if they have a prescription for the synthetic version of cannabis, known as Marinol (dronabinol), and they've purchased it pharmaceutically, and they test positive for cannabis, that's okay. The rationale is that medication was *prescribed* by a physician as opposed to *recommended* by a physician, and it was purchased in a pharmacy as opposed to a dispensary.

And regardless of any of this, please understand that *all cannabis that is used is medicinal.* It all works on those receptors we've discussed in this book. Those receptors are there, and regardless of what your condition is you are stimulating the endocannabinoid system and by doing so, it's affording you the opportunity and the ability to be healthy. So regardless of whether you participate recreationally or medicinally, you are going to benefit.

Again, things are changing. I was interviewed a few weeks ago for *Rolling Stone* magazine, an article to be published around the launch of this book, for their cannabis issue. The topic was cannabis and sports. Eye opening! It can be very eye opening, for example, to step inside the now recreation-legal dispensaries in any of the (currently) 10 states that allow recreational adult use. No more late-night parking lot deals. No more self-medicating like stabs in the dark. Florida Governor Ron DeSantis so far is 100 percent more open to medical cannabis than his predecessor. In fact when he took office he had a press conference in Orlando. Flanking him on one side was attorney John Morgan who had challenged the Florida legislature through a lawsuit to make *flower* available to medical cannabis patients, and it came through. Patients needed their medication.

It's my hope that the many families who have lived kind of underground can finally come out into the sunlight now, and it's getting better. You hear about people who secure cannabis illegally for a family member's Crohn's Disease, for example, who have been forced to make a choice—break the law and have a healthy, symptom-free solution to a terrible ailment, or watch your son suffer from either the disease itself or the dangerous side-effects of drugs. But today, thanks to recent changes in the law, that solution can be pursued legally, especially with a diagnoses such as Crohn's.

Are *you* or someone you love a potential cannabis patient? I'm passionate about cannabis because it is true medicine with zero side-effects. It doesn't get any better than that. Even water in excess has side-effects. Unless you end up "greening out," with momentary shortness of breath or a sense of paranoia, but none of those are that big of a deal.

One day, history will bear this all out, and the winners will be the patients, first and foremost.

ACKNOWLEDGEMENTS

THERE ARE CERTAIN people I wish to thank for contributions to either my own career as a physician, my involvement in the medical cannabis movement, the medical cannabis movement in Florida itself, to this book, and to my life in general. Without these outstanding people none of this would have been or would now be possible.

Thanks to Dr. Romero, my own former pediatrician who turned the table on me and gave me that ah-ha moment at the ripe, young age of three. Because of that, whenever I see a child or an adult who does not seem comfortable, I will often turn the table on them and ask, "Okay, if you were the doctor, what questions would you ask?" If I get pushback or resistance from someone it takes the wind out of the sails of their fear. With kids, I put the lab coat on them, I put the stethoscope around their neck, and I try to give them a sense of power in a situation where they often feel they have none.

To my dad, who passed away by suicide when I was 11 years old. He always encouraged me. My dad was a full-time x-ray technician at Memorial Sloan Kettering

Hospital in New York. He also worked part-time at another hospital and weekends performing mammograms at an OBGYN's office. Still, Saturdays were our days to be together. Saturday mornings I would go into work with him and he would put one of the white smocks on me and I would have that reinforcement, and Saturday afternoons were my days to hang out with my dad. We'd go to the movies, see a play, go to Madison Square Garden and watch the rodeo, or go ice skating together. He ascended from being an x-ray technician to radiation technician. In fact, he delivered the radiation treatments at Sloan Kettering to Brian Piccolo, the professional football player whose battle with brain cancer was documented in the movie *Brian's Song* with James Caan and Billy Dee Williams in the late 1960s. In 1972 my dad was admitted to the new pilot program for physician's assistants. He was a pioneer in his own right. It was the 1960s. Racial tensions were high. Hispanics were not well recognized. He wanted to be a physician but because he was Hispanic it didn't pan out for him. But he taught me my work ethic and about being passionate about your career, as he always was.

To attorney John Morgan and his brother Tim. Tim's tragic accident and neck injury as a young man left him in a wheelchair as a senior in high school. Today, all these years later, he and brother John are the biggest and most effective proponents for medical cannabis in Florida, to the benefit of so many. Had it not been for John Morgan's work, for his diligence, for putting his money where his mouth is, gathering awareness and support for the movement, none of this would have taken place and I would not be who I am.

To my patients, especially those first two cannabis patients, who allowed media into their lives. My first cannabis patient, (an adult female) found me through the list of certifying physicians in Florida. At the time there were still only about 30 of us. She called five offices and the first four were unprepared. But the fifth office was mine. I was in Orange City at the time and she called us from New Smyrna Beach. My staff already knew that I was moving in the direction of recommending medical cannabis, and when they brought her message to me I immediately told them, "Yes, set her up!" I was listed as the medical director in two of the regions Surterra Wellness (www.surterra.com) had applied for licensing in so I knew what the laws and regulations were going to be far sooner than anyone else. She came in to see me in the spring of 2016 and we began our doctor-patient relationship (a 90-day relationship was required prior to recommending cannabis). Once there was product available she became the first patient in Volusia County, in fact in the whole Central Florida area. As a result, I had every media outlet in my parking lot. There were so many reporters showing up the office could not contain all of them, much less all of their cameras and equipment. It was a zoo. The outside of the office was packed with TV crews and camera vans. Patients started texting me and trying to find out what was going on. "Watch the news tonight," I told them. And that was the first cannabis patient. The second was a little boy whose mother allowed for the media to go to their home, because that's where their treatment had been *donated* and delivered by Surterra Wellness. Those two events gave me the exposure and the wherewithal for people to find me, reach out to me, get seen, and get started on their journeys. I still have many of those initial people as patients today.

Thanks to Surterra Wellness, as the medical marijuana treatment center that was there and available to provide treatment to my first two patients. It was huge.

Grateful thanks of course to Professor Lumír Ondřej Hanuš. In addition to his pioneering discoveries in the field and his lifelong advocacy for responsible medical use of cannabis, his valuable contribution to this book and thereby our efforts in Florida and elsewhere cannot ever be overestimated.

And thanks as well to our beta readers: Christina Debusk, Deedee Diaz, Juan Jaramillo, and David Sacks, to name a few. From disparate fields and perspectives (a few previously in opposition) they brought fresh insight to the content and helped shape the book you now hold.

ABOUT THE
AUTHOR

Dr. Joseph Rosado, M.D.

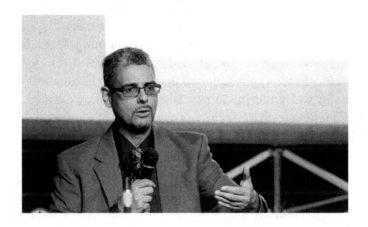

AFTER SPENDING SEVERAL YEARS in central Florida working as an orderly and then an EMT/Paramedic, Dr. Rosado realized his passion for the medical profession. He started chiropractic school at Life College in Marietta, Georgia, where he graduated cum laude with a Bachelor of Science degree in clinical nutrition and a Doctor of Chiropractic degree. After practicing for several years, he went on to Universidad Central del Este, in San Pedro de Macoris, Dominican Republic, where in 2001 he graduated summa cum laude with his medical degree. After working as physician and clinic Director in Salt Lake City, UT, team physician for the Costa Rican Institute of Recreation and Sports, and staff physician at Hospital Metropolitano in San Juan, PR,

Dr. Rosado relocated back to Florida. In 2005 Dr. Rosado completed his MBA in Health Care Management from University of Phoenix, magna cum laude. Once back in Florida, he worked as the Director of the Communicable Disease Division/Epidemiology and immunization departments as well as the Sr. Lead Physician at St. Johns County Health Department.

Dr. Rosado then moved on to Tricounty Hospital in Williston, FL to be the medical director, and also worked in a private practice with the Institute of Medical and Cardiovascular Excellence (IME/ICE) in Williston and The Villages providing primary and functional/regenerative care. Upon resigning from both Tricounty Hospital and ICE, he worked as a temporary (Locum Tenens) physician at the North FL Evaluation and Treatment Center in Gainesville, FL, Pinellas County Jail in Clearwater, FL, Escambia County Jail in Pensacola, FL, Florida Health Source in Pierson/Deland/Deltona, FL.

Presently, Dr. Rosado is the Medical Director at Coastal Wellness Centers in Ormond Beach, FL and is providing Therapeutic Cannabis (Medical Marijuana) recommendations and Suboxone Therapy; and volunteers once a month at Shepherd's Hope Community Clinic, in Longwood, FL.

He was on the bureau of speakers for the United For Care (Amendment 2) campaign in 2014 and 2016 and in 2015 Dr. Rosado took both the Florida Physicians Cannabis Course and the Florida Cannabis Medical Directors Course. In August of 2016, he was the first to recommend high-CBD/low-THC in the greater Central Florida region to an adult patient with Stage 3 brain cancer and in November of 2016, he was the first to recommend medical cannabis (THC:CBD 1:1), in the state of FL, to a pediatric patient, who was terminally ill. To date, he has worked with over 2,000 patients for the evaluation, recommendation and management of medical cannabis.

LEARN MORE

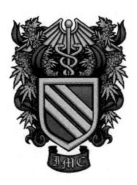

Are *you* or someone you love a potential cannabis patient and don't know if your condition qualifies for medical cannabis under Florida law?

Contact me today for a free consultation about your case.

Dr. Joseph Rosado, M.D.
www.JosephRosadoMD.com
info@josephrosadomd.com
1 (866) 763-7991

Dr. Rosado is also a well-known speaker in the field of cannabis advocacy and established medical cannabis consultant, training others in how to recommend medical cannabis. Book him as a speaker or discover his current training programs today!

INDEX

NOTES

Foreword by Professor Lumír Ondřej Hanuš

- Professor Lumír Ondřej Hanuš: (accessed 2018, December 14). *Prof. Lumir.* Retrieved from https://lumirlab.com/prof-lumir/

INTRODUCTION

- In a recent Medscape report: http://www.medscape.com/features/slideshow/lifestyle/2016/public/overview#page=1

PART I: CONTROVERSY

| 1 | Reefer Madness

- On his first: McWilliams, John C. (1990). *The Protectors: Anslinger and the Federal Bureau of Narcotics (1930–1962)*. University of Delaware Press.
- And he did: Rowe, Thomas C. (2006). "Federal narcotics laws and the war on drugs: money down a rat hole." Psychology Press.
- Up until 1910: (accessed 2018, July 22). *The Origin of the Word 'Marijuana.'* Retrieved from https://www.leafly.com/
- The rise of: (accessed 2018, July 22). *The Origin of the Word 'Marijuana.'* Retrieved from https://www.leafly.com/
- Anslinger also played: (accessed 2018, July 22). *Reefer Madness (1936)*. Retrieved from https://www.imdb.com/
- Today *Reefer Madness:* Murphy, Kevin; Studney, Dan. *The History of Reefer Madness*
- While Harry Anslinger: (accessed 2018, July 22). *The Origin of the Word 'Marijuana.'* Retrieved from https://www.leafly.com/
- Regardless of his inner beliefs: Wing, N. (2014, January 14). *Marijuana Prohibition Was Racist From The Start. Not*

Much Has Changed. Retrieved from
https://www.huffingtonpost.com/

[2] Tricky Dick

- From a recording: Posted by Loyola, C. (2014, April 7). *Nixon on who's really responsible for the marijuana epidemic.* Retrieved from https://www.youtube.com
- Perhaps Richard Nixon: Zeese, K. (2002, March 20). *Once-Secret "Nixon Tapes" Show Why the U.S. Outlawed Pot.* Retrieved from https://www.alternet.org/

[4] Social Stigmas

- JUDGE: "Do the defendants": From a recording: Posted by Nedd, A. (2016, August 31). *Gene Wilder in "The Producers" Final Scene.* Retrieved from https://www.youtube.com

PART II: SCIENCE

[5] What is Cannabis?

- A tall plant: Retrieved from:
  https://en.oxforddictionaries.com/definition/cannabis
- Cannabis is a genus: Guy, Geoffrey William; Brian Anthony Whittle; Philip Robson (2004). *The Medicinal Uses of Cannabis and Cannabinoids.* Pharmaceutical Press
- a tall Asian herb: Retrieved from https://www.merriam-webster.com/dictionary/cannabis
- the word 'Cannabis': Retrieved from:
  https://www.urbandictionary.com/define.php?term=Cannabis
- Hemp is a form of: Retrieved from
  https://www.britannica.com/plant/cannabis-plant
- By "hemp" we generally: (accessed 2018, September 20). *What is Hemp?* Retrieved from
  http://www.hemp.com/what-is-hemp/

[6] What is Hemp?

- There is often: Hogeye, B. (accessed 2018, September 21). *The Rise and Fall of Marijuana.* Retrieved from:
  http://www.ozarkia.net/bill/pot/RiseFallMarijuana.html

[7] Types of Cannabis

- That said, many recreational: (accessed 2018, September 18). *Marijuana stops child's severe seizures.* Retrieved from https://www.cnn.com/2013/08/07/health/charlotte-child-medical-marijuana/index.html

[8] How Does it Work?

- Through the ages: Retrieved from http://time.com/4298038/marijuana-history-in-america/
- Prohibition culminated in 1970: Retrieved from http://www.fda.gov/regulatoryinformation/legislation/ucm148726.htm
- Yet, despite its "illegal" status: Retrieved from https://moneymorning.com/2016/11/09/map-states-legalizing-marijuana-in-2017/
- Despite the long history: (accessed 2018, July 12). Retrieved from the video, "The Endocannabinoid System," https://www.youtube.com/watch?v=Z-OEpwgv6aM&feature=youtu.be
- And yes, you read that right: Sulak, D. *Introduction to the Endocannabinoid System.* (accessed 2015). Retrieved from http://norml.org/library/item/introduction-to-the-endocannabinoid-system
- Remember, endogenous cannabinoids: Pfrommer, R. *A beginner's guide to the endocannabinoid system: The reason our bodies so easily process cannabis.* (accessed 2015). Retrieved from http://reset.me/story/beginners-guide-to-the-endocannabinoid-system/
- And further, the endocannabinoid system: Miller LK, Devi LA. *The highs and lows of cannabinoid receptor expression in disease: mechanisms and their therapeutic implications.* Pharmacol Rev. 2011;63(3):461-470.
- Most cannabinoids: Jikomes, N. (accessed 2018, August 21). *List of Major Cannabinoids in Cannabis and Their Effects.* Retrieved from https://www.leafly.com/news/cannabis-101/list-major-cannabinoids-cannabis-effects
- This is found elsewhere: Herring, D. (accessed 2018, September 29). *Evolving in the Presence of Fire.* Retrieved from https://earthobservatory.nasa.gov/Features/BOREASFire
- And as most of us: Ukers, William Harrison (1922). "All About Coffee." *Tea and Coffee Trade Journal*

- Cannabis, like every other: Morgan, A. (2018, June 13). *What are Terpenes? Ask a 420 Tour Guide.* Retrieved from https://my420tours.com/what-are-terpenes/

[9] Benefits of Cannabinoids

- (list of ailments, cannabinoids, and benefits) Based on chart retrieved from https://www.leafly.com/

PART III: LAW

[10] Approved Diagnoses

- "I'm going to look at: "Morgan, whose younger brother was paralyzed at as teenage lifeguard after a diving accident, believes that smoking "is a medically effective and efficient way" to administer the active chemicals in cannabis for patients. He poured more than $4 million into the campaign to pass the amendment and is now bankrolling the lawsuit (to allow smoking for medical reasons)." — http://www.tampabay.com/florida-politics/buzz/2018/05/16/why-cant-patients-smoke-marijuana-in-florida-john-morgan-pushes-for-answers-today-in-court/
- For many years: (accessed 2018, August 9). Retrieved from http://www.floridahealth.gov/programs-and-services/office-of-medical-marijuana-use/_documents/ocu-timeline.pdf
- Florida started legalization: Thompson, M. (accessed 2018, September 15). *Senate Bill 1030 is a Go - Rick Scott Legalizes Medical Marijuana in Florida.* Retrieved from https://www.centralflalaw.com/senate-bill-1030-is-a-go-rick-scott-legalizes-medical-marijuana.html
- At this writing: (accessed 2018, August 9). Retrieved from https://www.flsenate.gov/Session/Bill/2017A/00008A
- Those diagnoses named: (accessed 2018, August 9). This is also an excellent infographic on what's covered as well as how to go about obtaining medical cannabis, by FloridaHealth.gov: https://floridahealthstory.org/stories/ommu-patients/index.html
- And while that's: ibid
- Foreseeing a "multibillion-dollar": Rosica, J. (2018, July 23). *Saying 'yes' to marijuana money, new bank comes to Florida.* Retrieved from

https://floridapolitics.com/archives/269356-marijuana-money-new-bank

[11] Becoming a Patient

- How do you become: Lewis, J. (accessed 2018, August 17). *Florida Governor Signs Medical Marijuana Law*. Retrieved from https://www.jdsupra.com/legalnews/florida-governor-signs-medical-39209/
- As of March 2017: (accessed 2018, June 13). Retrieved from http://www.floridahealth.gov/programs-and-services/office-of-medical-marijuana- use/registry-id-cards/index.html
- To apply to become: (accessed 2018). *Medical Marijuana Use Registry*. Retrieved from https://curegistry.flhealth.gov/
- To get your online application: (accessed 2018, September 21). Retrieved from http://www.floridahealth.gov/programs-and-services/office-of-medical-marijuana-use/registry-id- cards/index.html
- There's a valid argument:
  - Aggarwal, SK. *Cannabinergic pain medicine: a concise clinical primer and survey of randomized-controlled trial results.*
  - Clin J Pain. 2013;29(2):162-71.
  - Grant I, Atkinson JH, Gouaux B, Wilsey B. *Medical marijuana: clearing away the smoke.*
  - Open Neurol. 2012;6:18-25.
- Once absorbed, THC: Maykut, M. O. (1985). *Health consequences of acute and chronic marijuana use. Progress in Neuropsychopharmacology and Biological Psychiatry*, 9, 209-238.
- In comparing smoked versus vaporized:
  - Abrams DI, Vizoso HP, Shade SB, Jay C, Kelly ME, Benowitz NL. *Vaporization as a smokeless cannabis delivery system: a pilot study.*
  - Clin Pharmacol Ther. 2007;82(5):572-578.
  - Hazekamp A, Ruhaak R, Zuurman L, et al. *Evaluation of a vaporizing device (Volcano) for the pulmonary administration of tetrahydrocannabinol.*
  - J Pharm Sci. 2006;95(6):1308-1317.
- The bioavailability after oral ingestion:
  - Agurell, S., Halldin, M., Lindgren, J.-E., et al (1986) *Pharmacokinetics and metabolism of Δ 1-*

tetrahydrocannabinol and other cannabinoids with emphasis on man. Pharmacological Reviews, 38, 21-43.

    o   Maykut, M. O. (1985) *Health consequences of acute and chronic marijuana use. Progress in Neuropsychopharmacology and Biological Psychiatry, 9, 209-238.*

- Cannabinoids are highly hydrophobic:

    o   Huestis, M. A. (2007). *Human cannabinoid pharmacokinetics.* Chem.Biodivers. 4: 1770-1804.

    o   Valiveti, S., Hammell, D. C., Earles, D. C., and Stinchcomb, A. L. (2004). *Transdermal delivery of the synthetic cannabinoid WIN 55,212-2: in vitro/in vivo correlation.* Pharm.Res. 21: 1137-1145.

    o   Valiveti, S., Kiptoo, P. K., Hammell, D. C., and Stinchcomb, A. L. (2004). *Transdermal permeation of WIN 55,212-2 and CP 55,940 in human skin in vitro.* Int.J.Pharm. 278: 173-180.

- Cannabis is known to be consumed: Carter, G. T., Weydt, P., Kyashna-Tocha, M., and Abrams, D. I. (2004). *Medicinal cannabis: rational guidelines for dosing.* IDrugs. 7: 464- 470.

PART IV: HEALING

{ 1 } Cancer

- It made me feel like: Weintraub, K. (2018, January 21). *Cancer Patients Get Little Guidance from Doctors On Using Medical Marijuana.* Retrieved from https://www.npr.org/sections/health-shots/2018/01/21/578986845/cancer-patients-get-little-guidance-from-doctors-on-using-medical-marijuana
- There is a wealth of laboratory evidence: (2015, March 10). *How and Why Does Cannabis Kill Cancer? The Science Explained.* Retrieved from https://www.youtube.com/watch?v=e5xyUIzARbQ&feature=youtu.be
- When Kate Murphy was diagnosed: Weintraub, K. (2018, January 21). *Cancer Patients Get Little Guidance from Doctors On Using Medical Marijuana.* Retrieved from https://www.npr.org/sections/health-shots/2018/01/21/578986845/cancer-patients-get-little-guidance-from-doctors-on-using-medical-marijuana

{ 2 } Epilepsy and Seizures

- I didn't hear her laugh: Young, S. (2013, August 30).
  Marijuana stops child's severe seizures. Retrieved from
  https://www.cnn.com/2013/08/07/health/charlotte-child-
  medical-marijuana/index.html
- Seizures, by themselves: (Accessed 2018, 20 October).
  What Is Epilepsy? Retrieved from
  https://www.webmd.com/epilepsy/understanding-epilepsy-
  basics#1
- As far as drawbacks: (Accessed 2018, 20 October).
  Epilepsy Drugs to Treat Seizures. Retrieved from
  https://www.webmd.com/epilepsy/medications-treat-
  seizures#1
- You may have heard: Young, S. (2013, August 30).
  Marijuana stops child's severe seizures. Retrieved from
  https://www.cnn.com/2013/08/07/health/charlotte-child-
  medical-marijuana/index.html

{ 3 } Glaucoma

- I now vape for nearly instant: (2017, June 20). Medical
  Cannabis & Glaucoma: Erin's Story. Retrieved from
  https://leaflinelabs.com/patient-firsts/2017/6/20/medical-
  cannabis-glaucoma-erins-story
- Many people think: (Article reviewed 2015). *Facts About
  Glaucoma.* Retrieved from
  https://nei.nih.gov/health/glaucoma/glaucoma_facts
- The idea that cannabis can be:
  - Woodridge, E., Barton, S., Samuel, J., Osario, J.,
    Dougherty, A. and Holdcroft, A. (2005, April 20).
    "Cannabis use in HIV for pain and other medical
    symptoms." *Journal of Pain and Symptom
    Management*, 29(4), 358-67.
  - Ellis, R., Toperoff, W. Vaida, F., van den Brande,
    G., Gonzales, J., Gouaux, B., Bentley, H. and
    Atkinson, J. (2008, February) "Smoked Medicinal
    Cannabis for Neuropathic Pain in HIV: A
    Randomized, Crossover Clinical Trial."
    Neuropsychopharmacology. 34(3), 672-680.
  - Abrams, DI., Jay, CA., Shade, SB., Vizoso, H.,
    Reda, H., Press, S., Kelly, ME., Rowbotham, MC.
    and Petersen, KL. (2007, February). "Cannabis in
    painful HIV-associated sensory neuropathy: a

randomized placebo-controlled trial."
Neurology,68(7), 515-21.

- Erin Delaney suffered: (2017, June 20). *Medical Cannabis & Glaucoma: Erin's Story*. Retrieved from https://leaflinelabs.com/patient-firsts/2017/6/20/medical-cannabis-glaucoma-erins-story

{ 4 } HIV and AIDS

- In addition to the remarkable: Rahn, B. (2014, September 18). Cannabis and HIV/AIDS. Retrieved from https://www.leafly.com/news/health/cannabis-and-hivaids
- HIV, or human immunodeficiency virus: (Accessed 22 October 2018). *What Are HIV and AIDS?* Retrieved from https://www.hiv.gov/hiv-basics/overview/about-hiv-and-aids/what-are-hiv-and-aids
- The current and most: (Accessed 22 October 2018). *HIV Treatment Overview*. Retrieved from https://www.hiv.gov/hiv-basics/staying-in-hiv-care/hiv-treatment/hiv-treatment-overview
- While the side-effects of:
  - Woodridge, E., Barton, S., Samuel, J., Osario, J., Dougherty, A. and Holdcroft, A. (2005, April 20). *Cannabis use in HIV for pain and other medical symptoms. Journal of Pain and Symptom Management*, 29(4), 358-67.
  - Ellis, R., Toperoff, W. Vaida, F., van den Brande, G., Gonzales, J., Gouaux, B., Bentley, H. and Atkinson, J. (2008, February) "Smoked Medicinal Cannabis for Neuropathic Pain in HIV: A Randomized, Crossover Clinical Trial." *Neuropsychopharmacology*. 34(3), 672-680.
  - Abrams, DI., Jay, CA., Shade, SB., Vizoso, H., Reda, H., Press, S., Kelly, ME., Rowbotham, MC. and Petersen, KL. (2007, February). "Cannabis in painful HIV-associated sensory neuropathy: a randomized placebo-controlled trial." *Neurology*,68(7), 515-21.
- Medical cannabis also boosts:
  - Haney, M., Rabkin, J., Gunderson, E. and Foltin, RW. (2005, August). "Dronabinol and marijuana in HIV(+) marijuana smokers: acute effects on caloric intake and mood." *Psychopharmacology*, 181(1), 170-8.

- o Marcellin, F., Lions, C., Rosenthal, E., Roux, P., Sogni, P., Wittkop, L., Protopopescu, C., Spire, B., Salmon-Ceron, D., Dabis, F., Carrieri, M.P., for the HEPAVIH ANRS CO13 Study Group. (2016, April 13). "No significant effect of cannabis use on the count and percentage of circulating CD4 T-cells in HIV- HCV co-infected patients (ANRS CO13-HEPAVIH French cohort)." *Drug and Alcohol Review*, doi: 10.1111/dar.12398.
- While research surrounding:
  - o Costantino, CM., Gupta, A., Yewdall, A., Dale, B., Devi, L. and Chen, B. (2012) "Cannabinoid Receptor 2-Mediated Attentuation of CXCR4-Tropic HIV Infection in Primary CD4+ T Cells." *PLoS One*, 7(3), e33961.
  - o Molina, P. E., Amedee, A. M., LeCapitaine, N. J., Zabaleta, J., Mohan, M., Winsauer, P. J., Vande Stouwe, C., McGoey, R.R., Auten, M.W., LaMotte, L., Chandra, L.C., and Birke, L. L. (2014). "Modulation of Gut-Specific Mechanisms by Chronic Δ9-Tetrahydrocannabinol Administration in Male Rhesus Macaques Infected with Simian Immunodeficiency Virus: A Systems Biology Analysis." *AIDS Research and Human Retroviruses*, 30(6), 567-578. http://doi.org/10.1089/aid.2013.0182
- In the last few decades: Rahn, B. (2014, September 18). *Cannabis and HIV/AIDS*. Retrieved from https://www.leafly.com/news/health/cannabis-and-hivaids

{ 5 } PTSD

- The cannabis helps mute: Muller, R. Ph.D. (2017, December 14). *Medical Marijuana for PTSD?* Retrieved from https://www.psychologytoday.com/us/blog/talking-about-trauma/201712/medical-marijuana-ptsd
- In the past, terms like: Parekh, R., M.D., M.P.H. (Reviewed by, 2017, January) *What Is Posttraumatic Stress Disorder?* Retrieved from https://www.psychiatry.org/patients-families/ptsd/what-is-ptsd
- SSRI side-effects can include: (Accessed 18 October 2018). *Selective serotonin reuptake inhibitors (SSRIs)*. Retrieved from https://www.mayoclinic.org/diseases-conditions/depression/in-depth/ssris/art-20044825

- SNRI side-effects can include: Marks, L. (Accessed 18 October 2018). *What is an SNRI?* Retrieved from https://www.everydayhealth.com/snri/guide/
- Marijuana for Trauma: Muller, R. PhD. (2017, December 14). *Medical Marijuana for PTSD?* Retrieved from https://www.psychologytoday.com/us/blog/talking-about-trauma/201712/medical-marijuana-ptsd

{ 6 } ALS

- Cathy Jordan has consulted: (2018, January 25). *Why can't this ALS patient be allowed to smoke medical marijuana?* Retrieved from https://www.tampabay.com/florida-politics/buzz/2018/01/25/why-cant-this-als-patient-be-allowed-to-smoke-medical-marijuana/
- ALS, or amyotrophic lateral sclerosis: (Accessed 2018, 30 October). *What is ALS?* Retrieved from http://www.alsa.org/about-als/what-is-als.html
- ALS can be difficult: (Accessed 2018, 30 October). *Amyotrophic lateral sclerosis (ALS)*. Retrieved from https://www.mayoclinic.org/diseases-conditions/amyotrophic-lateral-sclerosis/diagnosis-treatment/drc-20354027
- Cathy Jordan of Parrish: (2018, January 25). *Why can't this ALS patient be allowed to smoke medical marijuana?* Retrieved from https://www.tampabay.com/florida-politics/buzz/2018/01/25/why-cant-this-als-patient-be-allowed-to-smoke-medical-marijuana/

{ 7 } Crohn's Disease

- I've talked to people: Cassata, C. (2017, October 31). *I'm 17, and Medical Marijuana Is Keeping Me Alive*. Retrieved from https://www.healthline.com/health/crohns-disease/medical-marijuana-keeping-me-alive#1
- Crohn's disease is an inflammation: (Accessed 2018, October 30). *Crohn's Disease Overview*. Retrieved from https://www.webmd.com/ibd-crohns-disease/crohns-disease/digestive-diseases-crohns-disease#1
- While much clinical research: (Accessed 2018, October, 18). *Medical Cannabis and IBD*. Retrieved from https://www.badgut.org/information-centre/a-z-digestive-topics/medical-marijuana-and-ibd/
- So it was with great interest: Cassata, C. (2017, October 31). *I'm 17, and Medical Marijuana Is Keeping Me Alive*.

Retrieved from https://www.healthline.com/health/crohns-disease/medical-marijuana-keeping-me-alive#1

{ 8 } Parkinson's Disease

- 1:37 p.m. Doctor: "The best way: Global Informer. (2017, February 24). *Man with severe Parkinson's disease tries Marijuana for the first time.* Retrieved from https://www.youtube.com/watch?v=pC17CaLU74I
- Parkinson's disease (PD) is a disorder: (Accessed 2018, October 18). *What is Parkinson's?* Retrieved from http://www.parkinson.org/understanding-parkinsons/what-is-parkinsons
- Side-effects of levodopa: (Accessed 2018, October 31). *Medications for Parkinson's Disease.* Retrieved from https://www.webmd.com/parkinsons-disease/guide/drug-treatments#1
- Researchers have shown enthusiasm: (Accessed 2018, October 31). *Medical Marijuana.* Retrieved from http://www.parkinson.org/understanding-parkinsons/treatment/complementary- treatment/medical-marijuana-and-parkinsons-disease
- The dialogue and description: (2016, December 3). *Ex-Cop Larry Smith Treats Parkinson's with Cannabis.* Retrieved from https://www.youtube.com/watch?v=ie5WXDlxPWo
- Larry Smith served as: (Accessed 2018, October 31). *About the Film.* Retrieved from http://ridewithlarrymovie.com

{ 9 } MS and Chronic Muscle Spasms

- I had severe excruciating pain: Craven, C. (2018, July 5). *Researchers Say Cannabis Can Benefit People with Multiple Sclerosis.* Retrieved from https://www.healthline.com/health-news/researchers-say-cannabis-can-benefit-people-with-multiple-sclerosis#1
- The human central nervous system: (Accessed 2018, October 31). *Common Questions.* Retrieved from https://msfocus.org/multiple-sclerosis-faqs.aspx
- While no two people will: (Accessed 2018, October 31). *MS Symptoms.* Retrieved from https://www.nationalmssociety.org/Symptoms-Diagnosis/MS-Symptoms
- Treatment, then, focuses: (Accessed 2018, October 31). *Multiple sclerosis.* Retrieved from

https://www.mayoclinic.org/diseases-conditions/multiple-sclerosis/diagnosis-treatment/drc-20350274

- Research is starting: (Accessed 2018, October 31). *Researchers Say Cannabis Can Benefit People with Multiple Sclerosis.* Retrieved form https://www.healthline.com/health-news/researchers-say-cannabis-can-benefit-people-with-multiple-sclerosis#1

"I find it quite ironic that the most dangerous thing about marijuana is getting caught with it."

—Bill Murray, Film Actor

CPSIA information can be obtained
at www.ICGtesting.com
Printed in the USA
LVHW010130120121
676047LV00006B/436